What People are Saying About

Getting Hit, Getting Up, Moving Beyond:
My Journey Through Brain Injury

In her inspiring book, Joanne models my favorite communication strategy—reframing—and shows how it can produce concrete results in a life. She explains how she escaped the default choice of embracing victimhood by continually reframing the obstacles she encountered. She uses her own experiences with a Traumatic Brain Injury (TBI), physical injury, and grief to show how she reframed even the most difficult of life's challenges, enabling her to become not a victim but the director of her own life. She is the perfect guide to anyone who seeks to join her in the ranks of the thrivers.

Sonja K. Foss, Ph.D.
Communication Professor, Department of
Communication—University of Colorado, Denver; author
of 20 books including *Contemporary Perspectives
on Rhetoric* and *Inviting Transformation*

Getting Hit, Getting Up, Moving Beyond by Joanne Cohen shows an intimate glimpse into the important discoveries of healing from multiple brain injuries. Reading Joanne's book is like having a personal coach by your side as she openly shares her fears, frustrations and eventual insights into the recovery process. Her book is intelligent and funny while demystifying the complex process of managing your symptoms, the people in your environment and your

emotions from what is known as *the invisible injury*. Joanne is a courageous soul on a harrowing journey.

Mary Ann Keatley Ph.D., CCC
Speech Language Pathologist and Board Certified
Neurotherapist, Co-Founder of the Brain Injury Hope
Foundation; co-author of *Understanding Mild Traumatic
Brain Injury (MTBI): An Insightful Guide to Symptoms,
Treatments and Redefining Recovery* and *Recovering
from Mild Traumatic Brain Injury: A Handbook of
Hope for Our Military Warriors and Their Families*

I met Joanne in 2007 at a Brain Injury Survivor's meeting, that she was facilitating. It was obvious then that she is passionate about helping people (like me) with brain injuries. As a brain injury survivor/thriver herself, she knows what she is talking about, as this book demonstrates. This well-written chronicle, a combination of both practical advice and spiritual musings, could serve as a How to Thrive after Brain Injury manual.

Doris Sanders, BA, MPA
BI survivor (12 brain injuries), BI coach, colleague, and friend

Joanne has shared her story in *Getting Hit, Getting Up, Moving Beyond: My Journey Through Brain Injury* to encourage others to find their path. She is a model for how to overcome adversity and start a new normal. She is never down. She is either up or getting up. I was Joanne's supervisor as she started a new career. Fortunately, she disclosed her disability and together we were able to create a position with the right amount of support and flexibility that benefitted the company and worked for Joanne. Joanne and I have continued to work together as partners at CTAT, LLC and co-leading the Brain Injury Hope Foundation, a non-profit foundation dedicated to giving hope and helping individuals with mild to moderate traumatic brain injuries. Through these adventures, I have learned a lot from Joanne and I am happy she chose to share it with the world. Resources like Mary Lou Acimovic's Limited Capacity Model as explained in the book as well as other tools, are extremely helpful to the person who has a Traumatic Brain Injury (TBI), family members and friends, partners/significant others, co-workers, professionals who serve the BI community and employers. If you need motivation, inspiration, and practical strategies and tips for life and life after brain injury, this book, part autobiography and part how to, is a must read!

Gayann Brandenburg, M.S., Managing Partner,
CTAT, LLC and President/Executive Director,
The Brain Injury Hope Foundation

Wow! What a fantastic read…. Almost a dozen years ago, I selected Joanne for an important corporate leadership development position. Over the past 40+ years, I have selected nearly 200 team members. Instantly, I knew there was something different about Joanne. No, it wasn't her TBI (which she disclosed later in our partnership). It was her chronic positivity! The truth about Joanne is that she taught me more about diversity than I thought possible.

Our differences complemented each other and together we partnered to move the organization beyond its present state. This book is a must read for anyone living a life of diverse ability (e.g. all of us). Thanks Joanne, for putting this resource out there in the Universe for all of us striving to thrive and for the gift of sharing your soul!

David W. Birks, B.S., M.S.,
Former Human Capital Management Director
Talent Management, Policy Studies, Inc.

Getting Hit, Getting Up, Moving Beyond is Joanne's story of succeeding over the years through great adversity. But this inspiring book is relevant not only to those in the brain injury community, but also to the rest of us. We can all learn how to positively approach challenges by applying the lessons that Joanne shares. We are so proud of our sister for having the ability and the courage to write this impressive book.

Steven Cohen, DVM and Debbie Cohen, MBA

I met Ms. Cohen when she was looking for legal representation for her three motor vehicle collisions, which caused multiple traumatic brain injuries (MBTI). I was privileged to represent her for her injuries. I was immediately blown away by the positivity that radiated from Ms. Cohen as well as her dedication to fairness and assisting others. Ms. Cohen has absolute faith in the good of humanity, a quality today that is difficult to find. She finds the good in every situation and is extremely effective as a writer, coach, and a trial consultant.

I would highly recommend Ms. Cohen's book, *Getting Hit, Getting Up, Moving Beyond: My Journey Through Brain Injury.* This is a book that is real, and that communicates the absolute truth of brain injury through the eyes of a survivor. I will provide this book to my MTBI clients and I will continue to introduce my clients to Ms. Cohen, as she is often a light in the dark as I have said before, when it comes to the stresses and chaos that Traumatic Brain Injury can cause.

Rebecca Albano, Esq.
Law Offices of Rebecca Albano, LLC

Traumatic Brain Injuries are as devastating as they are misunderstood by both the sufferer and by their family and friends. *Getting Hit* provides a glimpse of clarity into this otherwise murky realm. Joanne's story is a genuine, transparent articulation of her courageous struggle to survive and eventually thrive following multiple TBIs. From my perspective as a professional grief therapist, Joanne's journey has embodied the essence of overcoming the losses associated with TBI's. In this book, you, too, will gain insight and greater understanding of the importance of courage, support and self-acceptance in surviving a TBI.

Rita Coalson, MA, LPC, NCC

This book is a great tool to learn about the realities and the recovery process of a brain injury. Joanne's candid presentation of her accidents and recovery provides the reader with the experience and intensity of the psychological and physical impact of this condition. It changes your life. Through Joanne's experience, one learns the efforts and determination that is needed to work on your recovery. This book provides a clear step-by-step approach to understanding the grief process and the feelings of loss one faces as part of the recovery process. We need to treat ourselves with compassion when we experience a BI. This will give us the energy to continue to move forward. BI recovery is a life-long process.

As a Traumatic Brain Injury survivor, I wish that this book had been available in my early recovery. I learned that having bonds with many professionals, family members, friends and individuals who are also recovering from BI offers the clarity that one cannot recover alone. Sometimes it takes more energy than what we have to continue alone. The strength of all impacts the strength of one.

Jose Reyes, Ed.D, LPC

The compelling story of Joanne's journey as a brain injury survivor is both hopeful and helpful. From the beginning, her purpose for writing this book has been to share with others what she has learned about surviving and ultimately thriving on her own path to creating her new post-injury life. Her approach is personal, inspirational, practical, and most of all, honest.

Vicky Bradford, Ph.D.

Joanne Cohen provides a road map for anyone who is dealing with various kinds of the damage we can experience on this journey of life. This book is filled with inspiration, compassionate understanding and practical life lessons to share with fellows on the journey and the people who support and advocate for them. This is a handbook for thriving.

Joanne McLain, Ph.D., LPC, LAC

Joanne is one of the most authentic people I know; what you see is what you get. Her life's journey has brought her to us, and it has shaped her to be the woman she is today. Years ago, during a phone interview, I never would have guessed the horrific history, yet this yellow stickie professional was exactly what our team needed! Thanks to Joanne, I entered into OD and the Coaching profession. What an inspirational story!

Lisa Hulla, M.Ed.
Professional and Certified Professional Coach and
Organizational Development (OD) Specialist

I met Joanne Cohen through The Brain Injury Hope Foundation Survivors Series. The well-attended conference was an obvious indication of the need everyone had to receive the support in living with a Brain Injury (BI). Wanting to better understand all the aspects and challenges this brings to survivors and their loved ones was a reoccurring theme. Being with this community and sharing our stories has personally given me the support I so desperately needed during my healing path in coping with the results of my husband's brain injury. My husband's bicycle accident threw me into a whirlwind of unknown circumstances and my immediate response was to be there to handle whatever came my way. This wasn't the time to grieve even as emotionally distraught as I was. I had to be his voice and advocate in accessing the best care possible since he was unable to speak for himself during this critical time. I soon discovered that our healing journey was going to be a marathon, not a sprint and that I too had to take the time to nurture myself. Part of this self-care was to allow grief to surface and be present to it. Joanne lays out her healing journey so candidly in this book covering the many tools on how to better cope and overcome the challenges faced in having a brain injury and the impact it has on loved ones. This healing journey requires determination, courage, compassion, faith and support. Joanne has been exemplary in demonstrating what it is like to move from surviving to thriving. Joanne has my utmost admiration for living out this truth and sharing it with her tribe.

Iris Reyes, M.M.
Vocal Performance and Pedagogy, For the Voice Studio

If it weren't true, Joanne's story might come across as the script for an implausible movie titled, "Four Car Crashes and a Funeral." In reality, this book is about perseverance, tenacity, humility and humor in the face of circumstances that punch you in the gut and tempt you to give up.

I met Joanne in 2007—approximately ten years after her first accident in the Bahamas—as part of an executive leadership program she developed and ran for a company I'd recently joined. She was clearly someone at the top of her game, and I was thoroughly impressed with her work and the positive impact and influence she had across the company. We became friends and continue to collaborate on projects these many years later.

Joanne confided in me early on in our friendship about the brain injury she received in a terrible car accident years before and how much it changed her life. I recall being impressed by Joanne's resilience and self-awareness. But mostly I recall thinking, *Of course it was a cement truck. There's nothing half way about how Joanne does anything.*

It wasn't until Joanne's car was rear-ended three times over a four-month period in 2014 that I got a fuller understanding of how daunting her earlier recovery must have been or how hard she must have worked to resume a version of her earlier life—becoming the dynamic Joanne I met in 2007. And several years later when Roni died, I observed how significantly grief can tax an individual's brain and the adaptive skills he or she has developed to accommodate the differences caused by TBI.

That's why this book is so important. While well-meaning folks like myself can be empathetic and supportive to individuals who have TBI, we can't do what Joanne does here. By sharing her stories, insights and lessons learned—including some earned at the cost of adversity and the fear of stigma—Joanne gives others with TBI the gift of knowing they aren't alone, that what they're experiencing isn't unusual, and that there are mentors like her who offer guidance on their path forward.

James Dunn
Vice President, Marketing and Public Relations, MAXIMUS

A voice…a gift…sharing her most vulnerable moments while blending in sound tools and professional advice for others affected with a brain injury to help them find their own path and discovery. How refreshing in a world filled will social media perfection to read of blunders and dark days through a vulnerable voice that gifts remedies and compassionate advice for others affected with similar setbacks from a brain injury. I also found Joanne's 13 keys to re-empowerment practical and sound advice for anyone. Thank you for sharing your story of a crooked pathway into a wonderful deep life transformed and realigned in each chapter of you.

Linda Arnold, MA
Treasurer, Brain Injury Hope Foundation and
Financial Consultant, Abstract Insights

In the 25+ years that I've worked with people who have endured struggles after traumatic brain injury (TBI), this is one of the few narratives I've read that describes not only the tumult but the *triumph* of life after injury. As I watch Joanne in the Survivor Series discussions, I'm often amazed by how she connects with so many people at once, and in such supportive and empowering ways; her book helps the reader dig deeper into the sources of her strength but with a continuous message of hope, courage and patient resolve. I congratulate Joanne on bringing the same personality and optimism to the pages of this book that she brings to others in her life every day.

Kristi Staniszewski, PT,
CEO of O.T. Plus, Inc., a provider of care for people with traumatic brain and spinal injuries in Denver, Colorado

Getting Hit, Getting Up, Moving Beyond

My Journey Through Brain Injury

Joanne E. Cohen, MA, CBIS

CTAT, LLC
6732 West Coal Mine Avenue
Suite 227
Littleton, CO 80123
844-444-4522
ctat@ctatllc.com

Disclaimer: This book is not designed to replace a physician's independent judgment about the appropriateness or risks of a procedure or therapy for a given patient. Our purpose is to provide you with information and understanding that will help you make confident decisions about your life.

Editing, cover and interior book design by LTCMedia

Joanne's headshots by Carey Abraham

Library of Congress Control Number: 2019939679
ISBN: 978-1-7338397-0-9 (printed edition)
ISBN: 978-1-7338397-1-6 (eBook edition)

Printed in the United States of America

Dedication

Say not in grief, "she is no more,"
but live in thankfulness that she was.
Hebrew Proverb

I dedicate this book in memory of Cheryl F. "Roni" Baker (1946-2016) my beloved life partner of 21 years who left us too soon. Thank you for always being there, for meeting me and loving me knowing I had a brain injury; for staying with me after multiple brain injuries; for sharing a wonderful life; for all the fun and not so fun times; for the gift of your infectious laugh that touched everyone who knew and loved you; for being my very best friend and soulmate; for accepting that I am a woman of choice and we chose each other; for all the support with my business and former corporate positions, and for encouraging me throughout our life together to write this book. This one's for you!

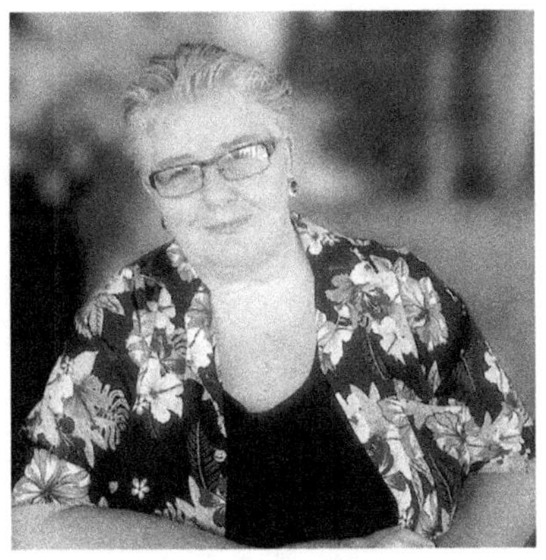

Roni Baker

I will love you always and forever.

Acknowledgements

There are so many people to acknowledge (many living and many who have passed on) during each stage of Getting Hit, Getting Up, Moving Beyond, and then Getting Hit Again and Again and Again as life happens—family, friends, colleagues, and practitioners. It is my hope that I remember everyone, and if I left anyone off this list, please forgive me. All of you have touched my life in some way, through some random act of kindness throughout this journey and each of you has made a difference in your own special way.

The brain injury community: You continue to touch my heart and soul and all who have volunteered and continue to volunteer for the Brain Injury Survivor Series, thank you! I would specifically like to thank Kristi Staniszewski, Barb Minden, Vicky Bradford, Lenka Karlikova, Rebecca Albano, Liz Somers, Dr. Jonell Perez, Dr. Shawn VanWinkle, Becky Miller, Liz Gardener, Alonda Martin, Doris Sanders, Julie Peters, Sue Fody, Christine David, Linda Arnold, and

Rena Thompson. In addition, thank you to all the practitioners who have volunteered throughout the years to participate on our Brain Injury Treatment Panels to share your valuable expertise with our community; Rocky Mountain Human Services and Carol McCright and her team for their support of our 2018 Survivor Series.

Family: My beloved Roni Baker; my Mom and Dad, Doris and Harvey Cohen; my brother and sister-in-law, Dr. Steve and Debbie Cohen; my business partner, Gayann Brandenburg (like family!); cousins: Shellie Levy and Kim VanCamp, Jacey Gordon, Sue Ellen and Ron Johnson, Doreen and Irv Shuldiner, Roger and Kaye Schindler, Babs Michael, Cheryl Berlow, David and Myra Berlowitz, Allan Shuldiner and Tawan Chang; my aunts and uncles; Jack Greenstein, "Big Sister" Sue Madison, Luanne Fine, Joanne Kipnes, Kathy Madison Penn, Lori and Ted Greenstein; my cats: Baxter, Moe, and now Brie Cohen-Baker.

Friends: Douglas Ray, Phyl and Terry Milway, Teri and Charles Steckly, Margie Elkind, David and Elaine Elkind, Linda Fankboner, Cindy Garcia; my Women's Group: June Clayton, Liz Gardener, Karen Karsh, Carol Hoskins, Vicky Bradford, Barbara Shor, and Avis Rich; my Geneva Group Spiritual Family (you know who you are); Melissa Teel, Sylvia Miller, Rick

Mueller, Terri Schroeder, Esther Davenport, Maria and Neil Cox, Janet and Pat Santaniello, Julie Peter, Sue Fody, Harriett Chesney and Brian Dillman, Joanne McLain, John and Sandy Ramirez, Doug Wills, Vik Ram, Darlene Tietz, Ronna Vigil, Sonja Foss, Susan Manfredi, Mark Perry, Lisa and Don Hulla, Michael Kilgore, Jonathan and Laurie Weiss, Glenn and Marian Head, Jill Patterson, Dr. Christine Daigler, Carol and Brent Hart, James Thacker, Xenti Hurst and Kathleen Colucci, Chris O'clock and Rick Chinberg, Craig Cellar, Mark Roncato and Bill DeMaio, Peggy Reed; my Survivor Series mentor, Nancy Freeman; Kim Gorgens, Debra Whitehead, Tyler Paris, Joe Lewis, my original CTAT team, Lena Beauchamp, Deb Stewart, Gwen Lawton, Clara Levison, Robin Harris, Mary Lea Cayer, Lynn Pollard, Ronald Precourt, Anthony Rodriguez, Diane Woodworth-Jordan, Gerry Schadegg, Marsha Dupris, Becky Miller, Lois and Arn Hart, Connie and Rob Stultz, Dorothy Thorngren, Lisa Kulp, Wendy Dinzl, Dena Mainord and Dana Brooks; all my wonderful neighbors: Ruth and Geoff Delin, Corliss and Mike Merrick, Mark and Judy Barnes, Sara Condoulis, Pam Cordeau, Margene DeYoung, Lois and Peter Florkey, Dave Gingerich and Linda Tobin, Fran Haefele, Ann and Roy Hager, Lisa and Richard Hendry, Loretta Leonardelli and Al Poe, Brian and Connie Nelson, Karen and Mike O'Meara,

Don and Susan Paladino, Sandra Tessier, Lynda Borel, Jack and Emma Romback, Joe and Lynda Feistner, Mary Jo Jensen, Jan Linquist, Nancy Hershner, Ginny Mayers, Judie Divita, Pat and Joe Oliver, and many more neighbors; friends at Lil Ricci's; Jesus Vasques, Carol Nadlonek, Melanie Mulhall, Brook Jasmine, Dr. Elaine Willis, Romy Leah, Goddesses from Maui Goddess Camp, Jane Evans, Belinda Waldron, Balancing Life's Issues (BLI), Ann Sheflin, Judy and Dave Feasby, Susie Crockett, Suzie Lambert, Susan Christe, Norm and Sheri Bell, Trail Daugherty, Roy Fawcett, Tom and Eunice Kinrade, Gail Davidson, Patti Cooke, Kathy Newell, Jill Bukowski, Robin Green, Rachel and Tom Claret, Karen Carrano, Jordyn Grote, Reina Kramer, DeAnna Bronson, Nancy Malick, Darla Coulston, Kim Tillotson, Sue and Mark Akins, Mark and Laura Lubline, Jen Scholfield, Lois Fink, Michelle Simonaitis, Jaimee Sodosky, Sigrid Farwell, Sotnik Weiss, and Amy Hoeye.

Fellow BI survivors and friends: Lenka Karlikova, Jeffrey Therrien, Doris Sanders, Liz Somers, Jay Clary, Deb Finegold, Bill Tassey, Colleen McMahon, Tina Garcia, Karen Hardison, and so many more.

Book Reviewers: Debbie Cohen, Jill Patterson, Gayann Brandenburg, Lisa Hulla, Sue Fody, Rita and

Jay Coalson (Chapter 7), Rebecca Albano (Chapter 6), Carey Abraham, and Jackie Lyndon Donovan.

Brain Injury Hope Foundation (BIHF) Current Board of Directors: Dr. Mary Ann Keatley, Gayann Brandenburg, Rebecca Albano, and Linda Arnold.

Thank you to all who have donated and given grants so we can continue to fulfill the mission of BIHF providing emergency funds and implementing our Survivor Series; Josh Meah (JoshMeah.com, LLC) for donating his organization to update our BIHF website.

MAXIMUS US Human Services: Kathy Kerr and her leadership team: Kelly Blaschke-Treharne, Laura Rosenak, Rick Sankey, Pat Aguilar, Doug Howard, Rachel Zietlow and others; James Dunn, Kim Colbeck, Melissa Janowski, Carolyn Abraham, Jackie Lyndon Donovan, and all the wonderful participants who attended classes and all coaching clients.

Former bosses who knew about my brain injury and gave so much support: David Birks (Policy Studies, Inc.) and Gayann Brandenburg (CTAT at Rocky Mountain Human Services).

Practitioners/My Support Team: Dr. Bill Borman, DC (Chiropractor); Mary Ann Keatley, Ph.D., CCC

(Cognitive Therapist); Nancy Bonifer, PT, DPT, MS (Neuro-Physical Therapist); Dr. Lynn F. Hellerstein, OD, FCOVD, FAAO (Developmental Optometrist); Beth Fishman McCaffrey, OTR, COVT (Vision Therapist); Amy Elsila, O.D.; Jenni Thune-Larsen, Optical Manager; Joy Zimmer, (Spiritual Intuitive); Victoria Atwell, (Bodyworker) and Michael Hegedus, (Bodyworker); Betsey Rise, (Weight Watchers Leader/Trainer); Dr. Brant Odland, (Primary Care Doctor, Kaiser); Rita Coalson, MA, LPC, NCC, (Grief Therapist); Rebecca Albano, Attorney; Nina Hart, (Hospice Affiliate); Kristen Burns, (Brain Trust Caseworker); Dr. Heidi Ray, (Kaiser Neurologist); Kelly Bastian and Care Team at Agape Hospice; Doctors and Staff at St. Luke's Cancer Blood Center (CBC); Dr. Jay Swartzwelter, DDS and his staff; Bruce R. Dunn, DDS and his staff; Dr. David M. Singer, DDS and his staff; Kimberly Gollick, RD; Dr. Paul and Hilde Wexler; Dr. Jan Lemon; and in the 1990s, Reverend June Kelly; Melanie Murphy, (Martial Arts Instructor); Deacon Dominic.

My co-authors for Chapter 6 and 7: Rebecca Albano, Esq. and Rita Coalson MA, LPC, NCC

Table of Contents

What People are Saying About 1

Dedication 15

Acknowledgements 17

Preface 29

Introduction 33

Chapter - 1 Getting Hit 35

Head on with a Cement Truck 37

Air Flight Angels 39

Surgery 42

Traction at Hotel St. Joe 44

A Story to Tell 54

My Physical Terrorist, I Mean Therapist 56

My Caregiver's Experience 61

A Victim of Circumstance 62

It's Just a Concussion 64

Lessons from Getting Hit 65

Chapter 2 - Getting Up **69**

Effects of a Closed-Head Brain Injury..................... 69

Music, Sound, Art, Light, and Other Therapies 71

I Found My Tribe 73

Letting Go of the Story... 74

Chapter 3 - 13 Keys to Re-Empowerment................**79**

Key 1 – You Are Not Your TBI 82

Key 2 – Focus on the *Ability* Not the *Dis*ability...... 94

Key 3 – Acknowledge the Small Steps...................... 99

Key 4 – Be Your Own Advocate and
               Be Resourceful.. 102

Key 5 – Consider Medical
               and Complementary Therapies 109

Key 6 – Develop a Support Team
               and Advocacy Network............................. 116

Key 7 – Move out of the Closet
               and into the World 119

Key 8 – Ask for Help 121

Key 9 – Compensate, Compensate,
    COMPENSATE!.. 123

Key 10 – Be Patient with Others Who
    Don't Understand 126

Key 11 - Know That Helping Others is
    Helping Yourself 130

Key 12 – Choose Your Journey, Your Life:
    Everything Happens for a Reason 134

Key 13 – Use Resiliency to Survive and Thrive....... 136

Chapter 4 - Maintaining a Career 141

The Good, Bad, Ugly, and Great........................... 143

Lessons Learned.. 147

Don't Give Up! 151

**Chapter 5 - Getting Hit Again and Again
    and AGAIN! 153**

Getting Hit Again.. 153

Getting Hit Again and Again................................. 156

Getting Hit Again and Again and Again 156

Chapter 6 - Navigating the Legal System 161

How to Select the Right Attorney for You.............. 162

The Insurance Assault 165

Process and Choices 167

The Litigation Process of an Injury Case 168

How to Prepare for a Deposition 172

Mediation 176

Trial 177

Lessons Learned Through the
School of Hard Knocks 179

An Outpouring of Emotions 181

Attorney Testimonial 188

Summary 190

**Chapter 7 - Overcoming Grief and Loss after
Getting Hit…Again!** **193**

Getting Hit AGAIN 193

What Is Grief 196

Characteristics of Grief 201

Grief Categories 202

A Grief Model 208

Styles of Grief 216

Self-Care Techniques 221

How to Help Others Support You with Your Brain Injury: A Baker's Dozen 227

A Final Note 230

Chapter - 8 Epilogue: Where I Am Today 233

Addendum 237

Joanne McLain Statement 237

Gayann Brandenburg Statement 243

Linda Fankboner Statement 245

James Dunn Statement 249

Roni Baker Statement 255

Extra Ordinary People 259

Endnotes 262

About the Author 263

Speaking, Coaching, and Training Engagements 267

Rave Reviews for Survivor Series 267

Rave Reviews for The Articulate Leader Program 268

Rave Reviews for Raising the Bar Workshops 270

Rave Reviews for Coaching 272

Contact Joanne 275

We encounter many defeats, but we

must not be defeated.

Maya Angelou

Preface

I've had a book inside me since I was 37 years old after I had a run-in with a cement truck while vacationing in the Bahamas. I also knew that I preferred to do many other things like speak publicly, participate on panels, be a keynote speaker at conferences, and coach people with brain injuries, especially as a trial coach/consultant. What brought me the most joy was being an integral part of the brain injury Survivor Series that impacts people who have experienced brain injury, the professionals who serve them, the family members, the caregivers, and their friends.

Writing a book was not in my plans, because as a brain injury survivor, speaking was far easier. However, when my partner of 21 years was diagnosed with leukemia and died in less than three months, a significant emotional event occurred that changed my life and perspective forever.

Going through that experience was profound, and I felt *compelled* to write this book. I did not want to suddenly exit this planet without writing about what I have learned about Traumatic Brain Injury over the last 27 years. The decision to write this book was announced at our February 2018 Survivor Series program, and I knew it was the right thing to do.

This book is intended to bring hope, courage, inspiration, help, and support to every person challenged with brain injury and those who surround them. For those without brain injuries, perhaps you will find something that will be helpful too, as life happens to all of us—getting hit, getting up, moving beyond.

This book is being published during my 65th birth year—an important and meaningful birthday for me and the perfect time to birth this baby!

This was not an easy process for me, I must admit. In fact, a friend, Julie Peter, shared a quote one day when I did not know how I was going to complete this commitment. The quote shifted everything for me and I moved on to finish writing this book.

There is nothing to writing.
All you do is sit down at a typewriter and bleed.
Author Unknown

Now that it is over, I can tell you that it was definitely worth the bleeding. It is my wish that you take from this book what will work for you and leave the rest behind. Every brain injury and every brain-injured person is unique with his/her own challenges and what works for me and for you may differ. So, take what you want and leave the rest.

A big shout out goes to co-author Rebecca Albano, Law Offices of Rebecca Albano, (Chapter 6) and Rita Coalson, AGAPE Hospice, (Chapter 7). Your professionalism, insights, and support while I was your client and then when we were co-authors will always be highly valued and appreciated. What you are offering the brain injury community through these chapters is outstanding and you have conveyed this information with integrity and from your hearts. Thank you.

Wishing you love, peace, healing energy, positivity, and whatever word resonates for you as you continue your life journey.

Joanne E. Cohen
May 19, 2019

Introduction

This is my message for anyone with a brain injury and anyone who is associated with or works with a person with a brain injury such as caregivers, family, friends, partners/significant others, and professionals who serve the brain injury community.

When I was 25 years old and a high school teacher in Elmira, New York, I almost drowned. I was sailing with some friends in Ithaca, New York when a gust of wind came up, the sheets cleated, and we were dumped into the extremely cold Cayuga Lake, where many people drown each year. A group of people who were in a boat race saw the four of us clinging onto two life preservers, left the race, and rescued us just in the nick of time. Hypothermia was setting in and it became harder and harder to tread water. While I was and still am an excellent swimmer, I honestly looked around at my surroundings, saw that it was too far to swim to shore, and thought we were all going to drown. The thought of letting go and disappearing into the depths of the chilling water almost seemed more peaceful than holding on.

Just then the race boat came up and they pulled us out of the water. They gave us dry clothes and took us back to their lake house to get warm. We were fortunate to be rescued. As I was warming up, I remember thinking that I must have more to do in life. This was my first memory of getting hit, getting up, and moving beyond, and I thought it would be my last. Little did I know what was ahead of me!

I have a plaque on my wall that says

God grant me the SERENITY
To accept the things I cannot change,
The COURAGE to change the things I can
And WISDOM to know the difference.

Chapter 1
Getting Hit

I haven't told the following story in years. I really did not want to revisit this very painful time in my life. I am telling this story now to provide a context for the remainder of the book. My intention in writing this book is to share with you the many lessons I learned from and because of this story.

My time on Great Exuma Island in the Bahamas was supposed to be a blissful escape to a beautiful oasis for a week. In hindsight I can see that my gut was telling me not to go. As a stress management consultant, I was teaching many classes on the subject for a major manufacturing company. In addition to the stresses of running my own business for the first time, I was burned out and desperately needed some time to relax and rejuvenate.

It was and has always been important to me to be a person with integrity—to walk and talk what I was teaching. In the middle of one of my workshops where I was training people how to manage their stress, I had a participant observer experience. I simultaneously experienced an outside perspective watching myself facilitating the workshop and an inside perspective listening to a voice in my head saying, *You are not being true to yourself. You are not walking your walk or talking your talk. Just look at your calendar! You are so stressed out. You have no business teaching this class. Accept your friends' invitation to go to the Bahamas. Take the week off to get your act together, then come back and continue the work.*

My friends had a second home on Great Exuma Island. They invited me to join them there. All along, my gut told me that I should not go, but my head told me to accept the invitation. I learned a long time ago, in Therapy 101 to follow my gut and trust my intuition; however, I listened to my head and on Tax Day, April 15, 1992, I left for the Bahamas. First, I flew to Miami and stayed overnight in a hotel so I could catch my flight the next morning to Great Exuma. I overslept that morning and almost missed my plane; another sign that I wasn't supposed to go. I was so late that all I had time to do was frantically brush my teeth and throw some clothes on before I left for the airport. Even though everything was telling me not to go, I got on that plane. When I arrived, my friend picked me up, and an unplanned journey was about to begin that would change my life forever.

Head on with a Cement Truck

My friend, Diane (her name is changed), picked me up in a little pickup truck that she borrowed from a neighbor, and we headed to a local place for lunch. After lunch, we drove to her vacation home. As we pulled

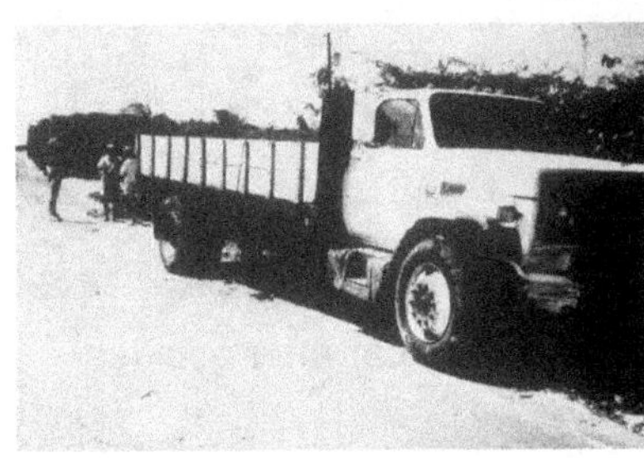

Head-on collision with this cement truck

up to the driveway, Diane's husband, Kirk (his name is changed), was dragging a branch toward the road. In the Bahamas, they drive on the left-hand side of the road; Diane pulled over to the right-hand side of the road to park in front of their home.

As I was waiting in the small pickup, suddenly, around the corner, came a big cement truck heading straight toward us going 65 miles per hour. Seconds later, the truck collided with the pickup, hitting us head on. To this day my mind replays the scene very slowly… I can see the truck coming at me in a rhythm–ba bum, ba bum, ba bum. I still wonder why I didn't just jump out. I later found out that the cement truck had faulty brakes, so it couldn't stop. Since Diane had stopped on the wrong side of the road, the pickup was lying directly in its path.

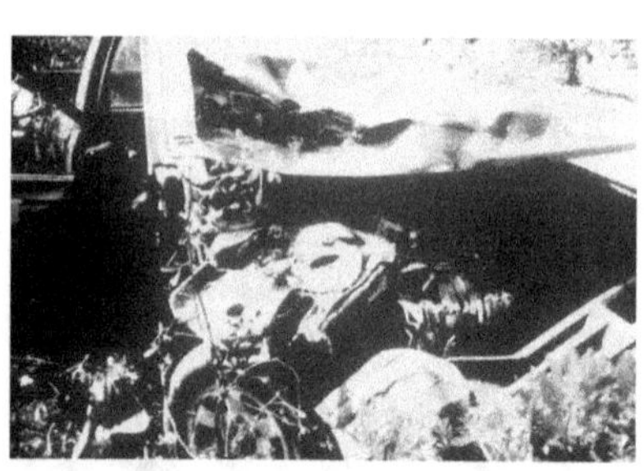

Crushed car after accident

I remember getting hit, but I do not remember the car spinning from the right-hand side of the road to the left-hand side. Only the truck driver and Kirk saw that. The next thing I knew, I was screaming in agony. Evidently, I had instinctively put my left leg up to protect myself, because my hip was pushed out of its socket and shattered due to the impact of the truck crashing into us. My nose was also broken. The surgeon later told me that it was one of the worst hip injuries he had seen.

People started coming out of nowhere to help. A doctor showed up and gave me some blue pills that did nothing. Some of the helpers ended up putting me in the back of another pickup truck and taking me to the airport to get me to a hospital in Nassau. I remember the agony of the terribly bumpy ride down dirt roads in the back of the truck. It was the most excruciating pain that I've ever experienced, and I wouldn't wish this pain on *anyone*.

Air Flight Angels

I had just signed up for a new insurance policy. Before I left home, I put the paperwork in my suitcase, took it out of my suitcase, and put it back in my suitcase several times thinking I would read it on the beach. Part of the policy was air ambulance coverage. I was self-employed at the time, so the extra $90 seemed like a lot. I remembered I had the policy with me, so my friends went through my suitcase and found it. Policy in hand, they made arrangements for me to be airlifted from Great Exuma to Doctor's Hospital in Nassau, about 130 miles away. I remember calling my best friends and my mother while I was lying there in excruciating pain. They were so upset and shocked to hear about my accident and how badly I was hurt.

At Doctor's Hospital, they put in a catheter; it took several painful attempts to keep it in. The doctors prescribed pain medications, but nothing worked. The room felt like a closet. Kirk found the paperwork and called an air ambulance to get me out of the Bahamas and home to a better hospital. I was too injured to fly commercially. I know how fortunate I was to have that air ambulance policy. After many long hours that felt like a lifetime, I was taken onto the air ambulance, a Learjet. The air ambulance picked me up, flew to Fort Lauderdale to fuel up, and proceeded to Denver, Colorado, for the next part of this journey—surgery and a *long* recovery.

I had my own nurse and paramedic while on the air ambulance. I asked the nurse to rub my feet, because it helped me to focus on something other than the pain. My medical team took great care of me. They saw my fragile condition. We refueled in Ft. Lauderdale and then proceeded to Denver. It was decided all along that it was best to take me home where I would have a better chance of healing. I am very grateful for that decision, because I ended up spending more than three weeks in St. Joseph's Hospital. Being close to family and friends during that time was a gift I will never forget. After refueling, we continued on to Stapleton Airport in Denver. Looking back, the ride on the Learjet would've been a fun adventure, like a *Star Wars* movie, if I hadn't been so injured.

That flight saved my life. I learned later that I had been in danger of losing too much blood from my shattered and dislocated hip. Ideally, I needed to get into surgery within twenty-four hours to stop the bleeding and get stabilized. All told, it took 24 hours and 30 minutes to get from Great Exuma to Nassau to Denver and into surgery.

The air ambulance cost $14,720, but when I offered to pay them as part of the insurance settlement, they would not take any money as their service was a part of my policy. I am forever thankful for those competent, loving individuals who helped me during one of the most challenging and painful times in my life.

That air ambulance policy protected me by providing a better way to get home versus flying commercially. I keep an air ambulance policy to this day and recommend it to anyone traveling.

When I was wheeled out of the ambulance, I was so relieved to see my mother and best friend who were waiting for me at the emergency room.

Surgery

When the stretcher was brought out of the ambulance at the emergency room of St. Joe's, my mother was waiting for me. I'm grateful I had the presence of mind to call her as I lay in bed at Doctor's Hospital in Nassau. One of my best friends had picked Mom up at the airport when she flew in from Sun City West, Arizona, and they were both waiting for me at the emergency room. The flight paramedic had called ahead and informed the hospital of my condition. I was immediately wheeled into the emergency room where I was moved, pushed and shoved into all kinds of painful positions in order to have yet another set of x-rays taken. Any movement with a shattered hip is unbearable. The first set of x-rays in the Bahamas 24 hours earlier were just as painful but they were not accepted at St. Joe's. Finally, I was wheeled into an operating room.

Lying on the hospital bed awaiting surgery, recovering from the pain of being moved from the ambulance stretcher to the hospital gurney to the X-ray table, I was scared. Then, I remembered what my father taught me when he was going through his cancer (what I call cancering) process: *Cohen blood is tough—I am not going to just lie down and give into this.* Those words were with me through my entire experience/recovery and have helped console me then and to this day. A nurse in a surgical mask looked at me with very kind eyes and told me exactly what was going to happen: They were going to administer medication and count, and then I'd go to sleep. She let me know that I was going to meet the surgical team and then be wheeled into surgery to repair my hip. I learned later that the surgery took over nine hours.

It was a very dangerous surgery, as it had been more than 24 hours after the injury, and I had major hip damage. As the nurse spoke, a sense of peacefulness came over me. I knew she was another angel sent to help me. To this day I wish I knew who she was, so I could give her a hug of gratitude. As I was wheeled into surgery, I said goodbye to my mother and my best friends who had rushed to the hospital to be there for me and for my mom. I thought, *If I don't come out of this risky surgery, I'm at peace and it'll be okay.* It was the first time I felt peaceful about my own death.

Traction at Hotel St. Joe

I spent three and a half weeks at what I jokingly called Hotel St. Joe's, because I was meant to be on vacation and the accident happened two hours into the trip. Today I have a six-inch plate, five screws, and a pin in my left hip. Fortunately, I survived the surgery! Two and a half weeks were spent in traction. It was agonizing.

Next up I had a year-long journey with physical therapy to learn to walk again. I didn't realize then that I had

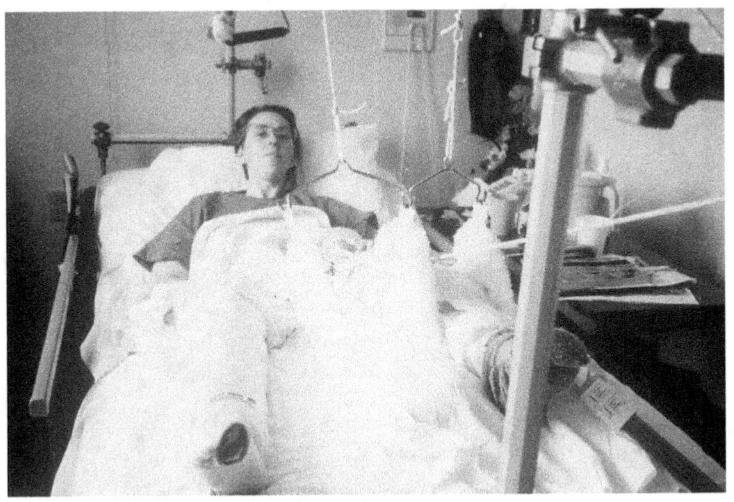

Traction after surgery

issues with my brain until I attempted to work months after my surgery. I did notice there was something wrong with my eyes—I was having double vision but didn't know then that this is one of the symptoms of traumatic brain injury (TBI).

Even though my gut had told me not to go to the Bahamas, I believe that no matter where I was on April 15, 1992, I would have been in some major accident. I believe this experience was a part of my path and my journey. It was supposed to happen because, in some way, I needed to go to the depths of despair, the deepest, darkest part of my soul, then come back

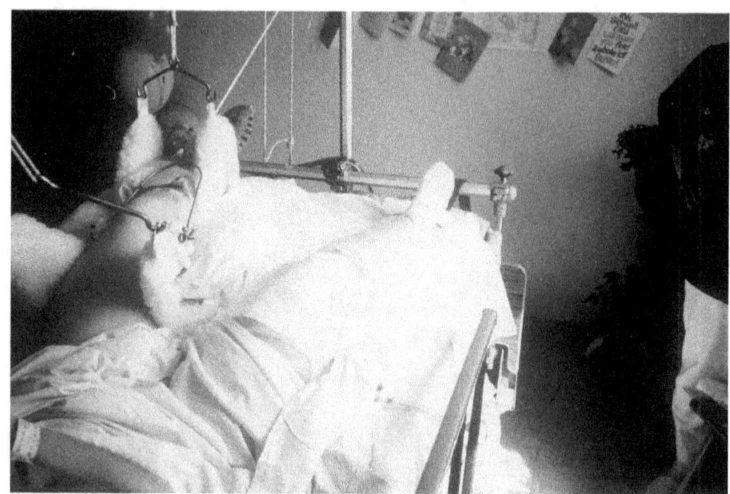

Metal rods through knee to stabalize the hip after surgery

to learn so many more of life's lessons. Now I ask for softer and gentler ways to learn these lessons!

The first two and a half weeks in the hospital were horrendous. In traction, I had a metal rod above my left knee from the left side to the right side. When I left the hospital, I was only able to bend my knee up to a 45-degree angle. After the first month of in-home physical therapy I was able to fully bend my knee. To this day, my knee does not feel the same; however, I am grateful to be alive and able to walk.

My hospital room was overflowing with gorgeous flower arrangements. I probably had over 100 arrangements. My mother had to start giving them away and let my thoughtful colleagues, friends, and relatives know that we did not have room for more flowers. My mom and my best friends, Margie and Phyl, were a wonderful support team. People just could not do enough for me. Because of the agony of being in traction, I had a Demerol pump that I could use every ten minutes. I had to be on heavy-duty medication for two and a half weeks until the doctor removed the metal rod. As I progressed, I switched to shots and then pills to endure the all-consuming pain until I got out of traction. After the rod was out, I switched to Advil, which continues to be my drug of choice for chronic body pain.

As I lay in bed with metal rods poking out of my jacked-up knee, I was comforted by the smell of flowers. At night, when I couldn't sleep because I was in so much pain, I would stare at the beautiful flower arrangements. The flowers brought such joy and beauty; they helped me focus outside of myself on things that made me feel good, displacing some of the pain.

There are many valuable lessons as a result of the accident. I am not sorry this experience happened. It taught me things I needed to learn, got me to engage in therapy, and actually led me into the brain injury field and soon become my calling. Until my accident I was so busy helping others that I never really understood how people viewed me, and it was quite humbling to see how much I was loved and soon became my calling.

While my hip was the most serious issue and the main focus of care while in the hospital, I was also noticing some unusual things going on with my eyes. At birth my eyes were not aligned straight. When I was three years old, I had two eye surgeries, and two more in the fifth and sixth grades to correct a vision problem. I went to vision therapy and had prisms in my glasses and graduated from this long process at 11 years old, only to be challenged, yet again, with some of the same issues at 37 years old and beyond. Just lying around in the hospital room gave me time to notice things and I knew something wasn't right with my eyes. I complained about this situation to the nurses several times, but no one responded. The crisis at the moment was my hip. I found out later how much our eyes are connected to our brain and how important it is to find an ophthalmologist who specializes in brain injury with the patience to work with the BI survivor to prescribe the correct lenses, prisms if necessary, and provide vision therapy.

I was a nice Jewish girl in a Catholic hospital with the Cross of Christ hanging on the wall in front me while confined to the traction unit on my hospital bed. People were putting my name in prayer chests. I was open to everything and anything that would help—Catholic prayer chests, Buddhist prayer beads, metaphysical churches, Jewish prayers, whatever.

Every day I focused on the Cross of Christ in front of me. Deacon Dominic became my friend and would regularly come visit my mother and me in the hospital room. He came, held my hand as the rod was removed from my knee and helped my mom and me in many ways. He was a true blessing. Firsthand, I experienced the truth that we are all one. It didn't matter that I was in a Catholic or a Presbyterian hospital, prayer was prayer, and I was receiving it from all over the country and from many religious and spiritual denominations.

Receiving or seeing angels in human form is an incredible experience. It is good to honor and respect whatever type of religion or spirituality someone practices; I believe we are all one and can support one another.

Hospital roommates came and went the three and a half weeks I was there. I saw people with bad hips and motorcycle injuries sent home very quickly. I was in traction and confined to my bed, unable to leave the hospital as quickly and so fortunate to have an insurance policy that let me stay.

I had only one bad experience at the hospital, a Nurse Ratched type experience (named for the heartless nurse in *One Flew over the Cuckoo's Nest* by Ken Kesey). My roommate at the time was in excruciating pain and Nurse Ratched yelled at her for asking for more medication. Then it became my turn to work with this nurse. There I was, an independent, strong-willed, stubborn, Taurus, career woman, lying in traction and completely vulnerable. I couldn't even wipe my own behind. On several occasions I felt emotional from the painful adjustment from independence to the vulnerability of not being able to take care of myself. I asked Nurse Ratched for another shot because I was in so much pain. She went away but did not come back. I waited a long time and when another nurse looked in on me, I told her that I was really in pain and had been waiting a long time for my medication. Evidently the other nurse was the manager and must have reprimanded Nurse Ratched, then Nurse Ratched returned, yelled at me, read me the riot act, turned me over, and angrily jabbed the shot into my derrière. The shot was extremely painful.

Being vulnerable and on medication significantly alters one's mental state. After seeing what this nurse did to all my roommates and how she administered my pain shot, I believed the woman had the capacity to kill me that night. She was my night nurse and I felt terrified of her, but I didn't say anything. I should have let the manager know of the situation; if I were in that same situation today, I would handle it very differently. However, when you are stripped of everything, even control of your own personal care, your whole life changes. There is a loss of the sense of who you are, vulnerability sets in, and self-esteem tumbles.

Life continued moving on as I lay there in that humiliating and vulnerable state. I was concerned about how to maintain my stress management workshops. I had several classes on the calendar but didn't know how I was going to fulfill my agreements. Some clients waited for me. Two colleagues, Gail and Carol, who watched and assisted me with my Performance Tuning: Turning Stress and Tension into Opportunity workshops, visited me at the hospital. We discussed how they could facilitate these accelerated learning training sessions in my absence. They agreed to conduct the workshops while I was recovering. While I was out of commission, my friends successfully took over the business for those clients who needed the training right away. I felt relieved that my clients could be taken care of by my colleagues while I did what I needed to do–recover.

When you think things can't go on without you, your ego is alive and well. I learned many life lessons during these weeks of being so vulnerable. One big lesson was the amazing capacity people have for compassion and love. Another was how to really receive. I had been a giver my whole life and now all I could do was receive, so I soaked it up. I received anyone who came to visit me with gratitude and joy. About two weeks into my traction incarceration a friend, Lynn, brought me a delicious pizza for dinner. It was the first non-hospital food I had eaten, and I was so thankful for that gift. It tasted better than any pizza I had ever eaten and was certainly better than the hospital food. It was a wonderful break, and I still remember how much I enjoyed that pizza. When I see this friend occasionally, we still talk about that moment and how appreciative I was then and will always be. It is the small things we do for one another that can make such a *big* difference.

On another occasion, my friend Linda brought me non-alcoholic champagne and chocolate from the Rocky Mountain Chocolate Factory along with two champagne glasses and said, "We are going to have a party!" I was still in traction and on pain drugs, so she made sure the nurses knew that it wasn't alcohol. We had a champagne-and-chocolate party, and I saw how happy people were while giving to me. I had learned how to surrender and lean into receiving, and it was an amazing life-changing experience.

When I had been released from traction, I was sitting in bed looking out the window at what appeared to be a beautiful day outside. The kindness of one nurse to bring a wheelchair and take me outside brings feelings of gratitude even today. The saying, *take time to smell the flowers* became very real that day. The sky was bluer, the sun was brighter, and the flowers and trees smelled fresh and alive. As I took it all in for 10 or 15 minutes, I felt like I was being reborn and saw the world in a new way. It motivated me to really want to be released from the hospital and go home. To this day, when I hear Louis Armstrong sing, "What a Wonderful World," I think about that special moment, and realize how it positively impacted my life.

A Story to Tell

I can recall that one day while lying in traction, Reverend June Kelly from the Boulder Church of Religious Science called me. After we talked a while I said, "When I get through this, I want to do a sermon about my participant observer perspective of the entire experience." She said, "You got it." I knew I had a long road ahead and I also knew that I was going to have something significant to say once I got through it all.

While lying in traction I didn't have anything better to do, so I began to take notes about the crash. At every phase of my recovery, I journaled my experience and what I was learning. I did my first speech, which was a sermon at the Boulder Church of Religious Science only eight months after the accident, just after I had stopped using my cane. I spoke about Getting Hit and Getting Up. That was an incredible experience with a 200-member congregation and many friends came to support me and hear what I had to share.

At the end of the sermon, many people came over to talk to me. Shanja Kirstann approached me and said, "I think I can help you." A few weeks later I started spiritual counseling with her. One of the things we focused on was my dreams. In 1993, we started a Dream Group of six to eight women. It was amazing work to analyze, explore, and discuss our dreams. Edgar Cayce, well known for his work about dreams, talked about an unanswered dream being like an unanswered message from God. The work we did together was powerful and many in the original group are still together meeting twice a month. I'm grateful to have this group of loving, supportive women still in my life 27 years later.

Another woman came up to me at the church after hearing me talk about living in the now moment as a human being vs. a human doing, and she gave me a *now watch* as a gift. When I looked at the face of the watch, instead of numbers, it said, "now" "now" "now" all around the clock. You can Google now watches and order one. I've actually recommended them to my clients, and they have benefited greatly by living in the present now moment. That watch meant so much to me—a touchstone for that period of time in my life.

My Physical Terrorist, I Mean Therapist

After a week of physical therapy in the hospital, I was released to go home. I had to be non-weight bearing on my left hip and leg for three months, so I was on crutches around the house and in a wheelchair everywhere else. Ed was my in-home physical therapist (PT) and was very good at his job. We arranged PT several times per week. At this point, I couldn't even move my hip an inch and could only move my knee to a 45-degree angle instead of a normal 120 degrees. Ed forced me to do painful exercises such as putting his foot in front of mine and telling me to push against it as hard as I could. Or pushing my knee into different angles, one degree at a time. My mother had to leave the house because she couldn't handle seeing me in such pain or tolerate the expletives coming from her daughter's mouth.

Four months after the surgery I was released to go swimming. I had a pool in the apartment complex where I was living at the time, so I asked Ed to bring his bathing suit and assist me in getting into the pool. This exercise became a huge part of my PT, as well as therapy for my mind and spirit. Swimming every day helped me through my recovery. I had to learn how to get in and out of the pool while on crutches. My friend, Douglas Ray, became my swim buddy. Douglas came over every day to swim and helped me lift weights. After Ed showed us how to get into the pool and we did some PT in the water, Douglas took over and we swam daily as part of my PT regimen. Ed showed me how to do the weights then Douglas took over as my daily PT partner. He came over to my home and helped me with the exercises that required assistance. I progressed from lying on the floor with a leg that I was unable to move up and down. Once we used weights increasing in increments of pounds, I could finally lift my leg using that left hip. When I started swimming, I couldn't even move my left leg an inch. Over the next few months, between the swimming and other PT exercises, I was able to put weight on my left leg and moved from non-weight bearing to weight bearing. Eventually, I was able to lift 30 pounds using my left leg, which was quite an amazing accomplishment!

My next PT was Mark, my external PT, whom I went to when I was able to drive to appointments. Unfortunately, my car had a manual transmission, so I had to borrow a friend's car. Eventually I sold my car and bought something I could actually drive. Mark was wonderful—he really understood the anatomy and physiology of my body. One day, he pushed my left leg (attached to my injured left hip) over to the right. I stared wide-eyed in disbelief at him and said, "That hurt." He didn't respond. I said, "Mark, don't you care? You hurt me!" His response was, "I am your physical terrorist—hate me now and love me later." While PT feels like physical torture, I learned that the more it hurt, the better I was going to get and the sooner I would be walking again. Looking back, it was worth going through all the physical therapy! Mark worked with me for an entire year, and I learned to walk without a limp.

During this time, handicapped accessible took on a whole new meaning. One of my first outings was going to the movies. My mom and my friend Margie took me in the wheelchair and off we went to see *Sister Act*, a movie starring Whoopi Goldberg. We parked in handicapped parking and used the space in the theatre to accommodate my wheelchair—both were a gift to me. Just going to the store for milk isn't an easy feat if you have to use a wheelchair or crutches. I gained a new appreciation for mobility during those months. To this day I get frustrated with anyone who parks in a handicapped spot when they do not need it. I needed the handicapped space just to get out of my car and walk to the store using crutches.

My living room was full of all kinds of physical therapy devices and equipment, some of which I still keep in my basement and loan out to others in need. I figured they would come in handy when I get into my eighties or nineties! The beautiful black-and-gold cane that I'm very proud of is ready and waiting for me when that day comes. I'm especially fond of that cane because I went from a wheelchair to crutches, to one crutch, to that cane in six months. It took another six months to walk without a limp, a total year-long recovery.

The day I walked without the cane for the first time, I walked into the doctor's office with such pride. The physician's assistant (PA) greeted me at the door. He knew how bad my injury was and how hard I'd been working. I proudly said, "Look at me!" I'll never forget his response: "Oh, you had a terrible injury, and you will have a limp for the rest of your life." I learned later that they had told my mother that I would not walk again without a limp or perhaps may not walk at all. She didn't want to discourage me, so she never told me. I was frustrated with the PA and felt angry at his negative response, and quickly responded, "That's not the truth about me."

After he made that comment, I came home and had a poor me pity party. I ate an entire box of Entenmann's chocolate-chip cookies. Then I called my PT, Mark, and while still in tears told him that the physician assistant thought I'd have a limp my whole life. He said, "I don't buy it, get back in here." We worked another grueling six months on the gluteus medius and gluteus maximus and whatever other muscles live in that vicinity. I even lifted 30 pounds of weight using the left leg and hip! While the physician assistant felt he was telling his truth, it motivated me to action: *I'll show you.*

My Caregiver's Experience

For my mother, the whole experience was devastating. I could have died from the accident, the injury, or the surgery, and she came and took care of me. She was very upset about all the pain and suffering I was enduring. After five weeks I thought it would be best for mom to go home as I thought I could do this on my own. After all, I had a reacher—a sock putter-on-er—and the bench for the bathtub. I had learned how to do many things for myself with the help of occupational therapy, as well as an organization that specialized in occupational and physical therapy, O.T. Plus. Sometimes it took every ounce of energy just to get out of bed, get in the shower, and get dressed. I would go into the living room exhausted, and that amount was all I could do for that day.

When my friend and I took my mom to the airport only five weeks after my accident, I felt emotional during the entire trip home. I wanted to be a strong, independent person and do everything for myself, but I still needed help. I sent her home a little too soon. Clients and friends who heard about my accident took me to the store and ran other errands for me; it felt like people couldn't do enough to help me, and I am forever appreciative to my mom and my friends.

A Victim of Circumstance

One of the activities I wanted to do the most was simply walk. Cheesman Park in Denver was right across the street from my apartment and I would sit looking longingly out the window where I used to briskly walk the path. At that point, all I could do was sit in my living room, watch people walk, and say to myself, *Someday that's going to be me.* When I progressed through therapy to crutches, I walked from my apartment across the street to the park and back and considered that a great accomplishment. Eventually, I reached a milestone goal and made it all the way around the park. To paraphrase Neil Armstrong, "One small step for a woman, one giant leap for womankind!"

Still, I felt a bit vulnerable in that park because I couldn't run if I had to. So, when I retired the crutches, I took a course in Boulder called Way of the Crane Martial Arts and Streetwize Self Defense.[1] In my injured state, taking this course was a bit scary. We had to put orange tape on my left hip because people would throw us on the floor during an attack scenario, and they had to be very careful with me. The instructors were not easy on me in any other way. I took that course so that if I was in Cheesman Park or anywhere else and someone came after me, I would not have to feel vulnerable anymore. I could take care of myself.

Taking this course was very empowering. One of the exercises was to write on a wooden board all the things we each wanted to release and let go. Then, no longer a vulnerable victim, I broke the board with my left foot. I found that board in my garage a few months ago. I wasn't one to be a victim in everyday life, however I was a victim of a circumstance.

It's Just a Concussion

Many months later and during one of my follow up appointments, I explained to my doctor that I was trying to teach a class on stress management at a major manufacturing company in Northern Colorado and had to have my friends take over because I could only last about an hour. There were times when I would be talking and suddenly not know where I was or where I was going in the presentation. Using music was good compensation. While it helped anchor me and trigger my memory, it wasn't enough.

When I told him all the strange things that were happening, he said, "Oh, don't worry about it, it is just post-traumatic stress; your brain is healing from the concussion, it will go away." Well, it did not go away! This was in 1992, when discussions about brain injuries were not as common as they are today.

Lessons from Getting Hit

In my first six months I went from wheelchair to crutches, and crutches to cane. I owe a large part of my recovery to my physical therapist and to my friend, neighbor, and colleague, Douglas, who spent hours each day helping me with PT exercises as well as swimming with me.

After 10 months, I facilitated a program for the American Society for Training and Development (ASTD.) This program consisted of a panel to discuss the Americans with Disabilities Act (ADA). I was still getting around using my cane, and I was motivated to get back into my professional life, one step at a time! This was the first work I planned and accomplished since the accident. It focused on ADA and people with disabilities (of which I was now a member) and it gave me a goal to strive toward and a sense of purpose and meaning at that time in my life. It was a forward step toward getting back to doing something—some sort of work. It was relevant and made me feel somewhat relevant.

Looking back, there were so many lessons that revealed themselves throughout this initial part of my journey. I learned the following from getting hit:

- Listen to your intuition/gut. It gives you powerful messages.

- Seek out the valuable lessons that emerge, embrace them, learn from them, and be open to them.

- Allow yourself to be vulnerable, without judgment, and trust where that takes you.

- To receive help and support is to truly give to those providing that help and support.

- Life throws us curveballs and opportunities. Our journey is shaped by how we handle what is thrown our way when we get hit.

My body was healing, but my journey with a TBI had just begun.

The best way out is always through.

Robert Frost

Chapter 2 - Getting Up
Effects of a Closed-Head Brain Injury

No doubt many with a Traumatic Brain Injury (TBI) have had similar experiences. I would be in a training session and talking right on point, when suddenly, I'd forget where I was. It was like the computer in my brain just shut down—a brain freeze. I didn't know where I was in my speech or where I was intending to go. I always used a flip chart in my stress management presentations. I could access my long-term memory and see three of the things from the flip chart, but I couldn't, for the life of me, remember the other three until 3:00 a.m. or so, lying in bed in the middle of the night. When my brain was resting, the ideas would finally pop back into my head.

During the first two years, I didn't know what was wrong with me. My doctor just told me not to worry about it. He would tell me, "You have a concussion. You have post-traumatic stress. It will get better," and I'd go home. Well, it didn't get better. I did my best to keep myself upbeat and positive for 10 months and then went into a downward spiral. It finally hit me. It was the first time I experienced feeling like I was in a deep black hole. I had the feeling of not wanting to be here.

Not knowing why I wasn't fully functioning, I felt very depressed until one day I got a call from the daughter of my dear friend, Phyl Milway. Her daughter, Teri, was working at Spalding Rehabilitation in Denver, and Phyl had told her my story. Teri called me and said, "You're not crazy, and you're not making this up. You have a closed-head brain injury." She explained that when the cement truck hit me head on at 65 mph, my brain, like Jell-O, was moved forward and backward, causing damage to the brain matter (this is called a coup contrecoup injury). I immediately thought, Hallelujah! At least I know what has been happening with me. Now I can figure out what to do about it. So that's what I did. For that gift of knowledge, my speeches have often been dedicated to Phyl, who passed away in 2012, and I will always be appreciative of her daughter, Teri. Phyl stood by me when others did *not* understand me and some friends even left me. Her guidance and support was and will always be valued and appreciated.

Today, we hear a lot of stories about head injuries of combat veterans, football players, and children, but in 1992, it wasn't even a conversation. Resources were not as well known or accessible at that time, so I went on a journey to search how I could advocate for and heal myself. I found some computer-type training programs that helped re-train the brain, but at the time I did not feel like I wanted to work with computers and technology. Then I discovered the Tomatis Method, recommended by Shanja, my spiritual teacher.

Music, Sound, Art, Light, and Other Therapies

I knew I loved music and art. I thought the Tomatis Method, a sound therapy program that uses the music of Mozart in addition to artwork, was the one for me! The music was increased to higher and higher frequencies until it almost drove me crazy. I created artwork that I saved as it depicted my journey. The psychologist who ran the program, Dr. Ron Minson, would look at the artwork, ask questions, and record my progress at each juncture. He observed my gradual improvement through my art, which went from inner agitation and anger to peace, love, and hearts. I was grateful to have the opportunity to experience this sound therapy program with the hopes of improving my memory and building new brain connections.

The next therapy recommended was a program called The David. This was a light therapy program that was very pleasant because I love colorful lights. I would lie down in a comfortable chair in a dark room while lights were being flashed by the technician. The goal was to boost mood and mental performance. I trusted the process and felt a sense of calm although I did not know how it was helping me. I just trusted the process.

I also worked diligently with my clinical therapist and my spiritual teacher. It was a very painful experience at this time in my journey. In time I rose from a deep dark place like the rising of the phoenix, a symbol of transformation from grief. Both the therapist and the spiritual teacher openly supported me, so I could go deep into my feelings. I trusted both of these therapists as they created a safe space. That allowed me to delve into my feelings of depression, deeply grieve the loss of who I was and the life I had before the accident, and to be open to my new life. I wanted to feel my emotions and move through them. I gradually rose from the ashes of grief and found purpose again.

I Found My Tribe

In 2004, one of my colleagues designed and facilitated a program for Denver Options (later called Rocky Mountain Human Services) called the Survivor Series, for brain injury survivors and the brain injury community. When she was diagnosed with cancer and was undergoing chemotherapy treatments in 2010, another colleague on the team who knew about my brain injury asked whether I could possibly cover for her and speak to this audience. I was asked to develop a presentation, and that was the beginning of being a significant part of the brain injury world. At that time, I was employed in a corporate environment, and when I spoke at this forum to an audience with brain injuries, I felt like I was at home. I knew I was there to help other people, and that knowing actually helped me. It took 18 years, and I finally found my people, my community, my tribe. I did not have to be perfect like I felt I had to be in the corporate arena. If I forgot where I was in my thought process/presentation, it did not matter. If I was having a moment, we would laugh *with* each other. It was an epiphany to show up and do something to support others and realize how much I too needed and deeply appreciated the experience and the connections.

Letting Go of the Story

I told the story, Getting Hit and Getting Up, hundreds of times. I was scheduled to speak at a Win-Win Business Forum in Boulder. The night before, I had a session with Shanja, my spiritual teacher. I will never forget that encounter, because she told me that I was stuck in my story. And it was true. Initially telling my story was healing; however, there comes a time when you and everyone else are bored with it ad nauseum. Re-living the accident over and over again kept me from moving forward. Shanja gave me a kick in the rear-end and I felt upset all the way home. This was an instrumental part of Getting Up *and* the beginning of Moving Beyond!

That night, I took the speech that was basically the story and rewrote it to focus on what I learned from my story. The next morning, I drove back to Boulder. I stood in front of the audience with my prior speech on index cards, ready with a brand-new presentation, Getting Hit, Getting Up, and Moving Beyond. I said to the audience staring back at me, "You don't really need to know or really want to know all the guts and glory of what happened to me, do you? I am just going to share with you what I learned from the whole ordeal." I threw all of my index cards from the initial presentation, Getting Hit and Getting Up onto the floor—this action had quite a powerful reaction and made an impact on the crowd and created a positive transformational shift for me, too. The rest of the presentation focused on Moving Beyond and lessons learned. Shanja was spot on!

While it was not my idea of a good time in 1992, I am grateful for that truck in the Bahamas, because without that accident, I would not have written this book, I would not have been actively involved in the brain injury field and community, and I would not have found my calling and an additional passion to pursue. The lesson is that whenever something negative or challenging happens in my life, I've learned to ask myself, *What have I learned, and how can I assist/help others with the wisdom gained from it?* For that, I am extremely grateful that I got hit and through much hard work, effort, positive attitude, support from family, friends, colleagues, and professionals, I was able to *get up*.

*Life is 10% what happens to you
and 90% how you react to it.*
Charles R. Swindoll

Chapter 3
13 Keys to Re-Empowerment

I have been speaking since 1992 about lessons learned from the accident in the Bahamas. My first speech, only seven months after the accident, was entitled, Getting Hit and Getting Up. As I progressed through this journey, so did my presentations, and eventually they became, Getting Hit, Getting Up, Moving Beyond: 13 Keys to Re-empowerment for Brain Injury Survivors. I also added one for professionals who serve the brain injury community and entitled it: Something that Matters: Getting Hit, Getting Up, Moving Beyond, and Making a Difference.

Adversity is something we all face in our lifetime. Getting through the situation is first and foremost. We can then ask ourselves, *What is the reason this happened, what am I supposed to do with it, and how can I help and support others?* The purpose of these presentations was and still is to demonstrate and encourage commitment to living one's life to the fullest as a new and different you. It is to also educate and share insights with professionals who will be or are working with brain injury (BI) / post-traumatic stress (PTS) / post-traumatic stress disorder (PTSD) and survivors who are coping with cognitive and other changes, challenges, and difficulties.

The following are 13 Keys that I have learned along the way to support the road to recovery for anyone who has been hit. What is interesting is the keys have not changed. What has changed throughout the years is what I say about each key, depending upon where I have personally been on my own road to recovery and what I continue to learn from others—an on-going process.

Remember, please take what will work for you and leave what does not. These keys were pivotal in helping me on my journey, and I believe we are all works in progress. Life throws us curveballs, and what we choose to *do* with those situations *is* something that matters. All brain injuries are unique, so some keys may be more applicable to you now, and others may help you later on in your own personal journey.

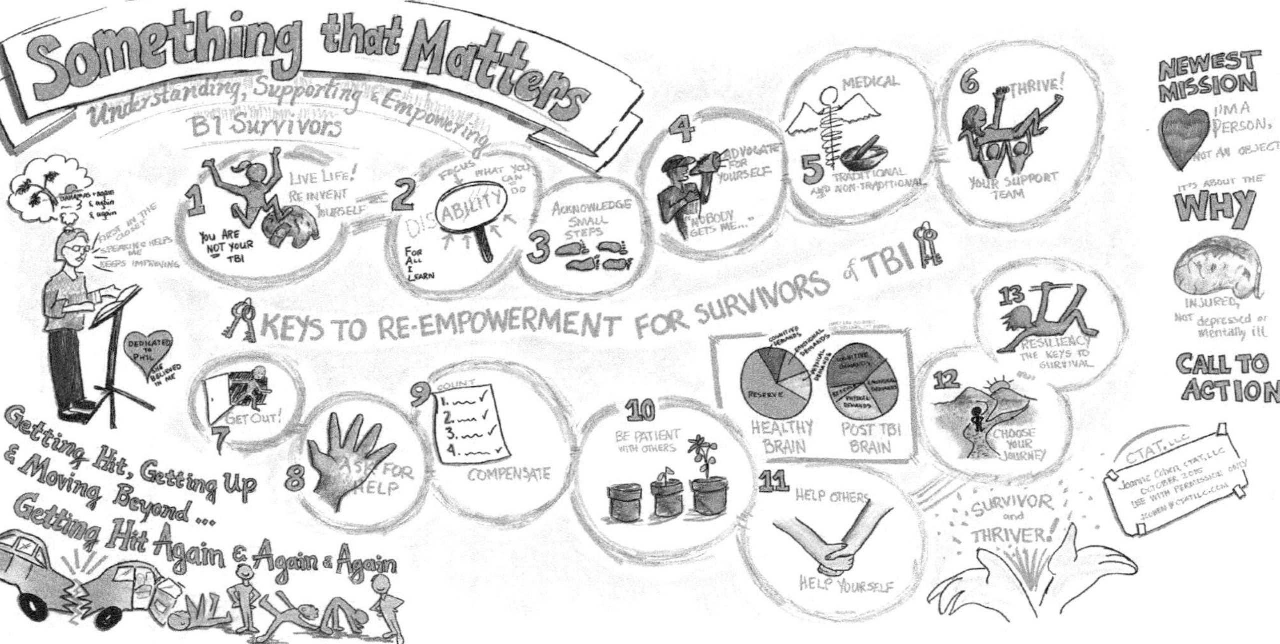

Something that Matters
Understanding, Supporting & Empowering
TBI Survivors
NEWEST MISSION
I'M A PERSON, NOT AN OBJECT
WHY
IT'S ABOUT THE
INJURED, NOT depressed or mentally ill
CALL TO ACTION
CTAT, LLC
ICONIC COMIC CHAT, LLC
COLORED ZONES
USE WITH PERMISSION
LICENSED BY CTAT, LLC, CCA, CAA
9 KEYS TO RE-EMPOWERMENT FOR SURVIVORS
of TBI
1 YOU ARE NOT YOUR TBI
LIVE LIFE!
RE-INVENT YOURSELF
2 DISABILITY
FOCUS WHAT YOU CAN DO
FOR ALL I LEARN
3 ACKNOWLEDGE SMALL STEPS
4 ADVOCATE FOR YOURSELF
"NOBODY GETS ME..."
5 MEDICAL
TRADITIONAL AND NON-TRADITIONAL
6 THRIVE!
YOUR SUPPORT TEAM
8 GET OUT!
ASK FOR HELP
9 COUNT
1. 2. 3. 4.
COMPENSATE
10 BE PATIENT WITH OTHERS
11 HELP OTHER
HELP YOURSELF
HEALTHY BRAIN
RESERVE
POST TBI BRAIN
12 CHOOSE YOUR JOURNEY
SURVIVOR and THRIVER!
13 RESILIENCY
THE KEYS TO SURVIVAL
Getting Hit, Getting Up & Moving Beyond ...
Getting Hit Again & Again & Again & Again
DEDICATED TO...
RELEASED FOR ME
Sue Teeby   www.sueteeby.com

I retained a colleague, Sue Fody from Got It! Learning Designs, to observe my presentations and create this graphic recording on page 81, an effective training tool that summarizes the 13 Keys to Re-empowerment.

Key 1 – You Are Not Your TBI

The first key to re-empowerment is you are not your Traumatic Brain Injury (TBI) so live your life to the fullest as the new and different you. Another brain-injured person once said to me, "I'm a person with a brain injury; I'm not a brain-injured person." Those are powerful words. Right then I decided that was how I was going to view my own brain injury. Understanding the difference lies in the power of our words. Our words affect our thoughts, and our thoughts affect our actions. What words do you use to define yourself?

The Broken Brain series by Dr. Mark Hyman has many helpful insights and important leading-edge information; however, the term *broken brain* does not personally resonate with me. I know that marketing a series called the Broken Brain can lead people to believe that if you have a broken brain, you can fix it.

For me, the title has a negative connotation and could make one feel like a victim. I will, however, own that I am a person with a brain injury. I will share that I have my challenges. I am also a professional with a brain injury who wants to help people with brain injuries learn how to move from surviving to thriving.

A Victim of Circumstance

To some people, a traumatic brain injury becomes their identity. When I was in the hospital for three and a half weeks, I stepped outside myself and viewed the situation from the perspective of an observer. I watched myself as I went through the process. I had to come to terms with the concept of myself in this new situation. Since then, I have overcome many obstacles and exceeded the limits of medical diagnosis.

I had to believe that I was a victim of a circumstance, not that I was a victim. While I may have felt like a victim initially, I had to rephrase/reframe it so I could heal. Many people I have encountered say they want their old life back. The truth is, this *is* our life now. Life with a brain injury is different, and it is one to embrace. It is a journey to face and work toward a new normal. Acknowledge small improvements. We can focus on memory loss, brain fog, irritability, fatigue, vision problems, light sensitivity, etc., or we can focus on what we can do about these issues as they arise. We can figure out how to move ourselves to the next level of improvement. If you do a reframe, you will begin to look at yourself as a person with a brain injury, not a brain-injured person. It's a way of holding a view of the glass half full rather than half empty. You too are not a victim—you are a victim of a circumstance. If you stay focused on being a victim, it may be a self-imposed challenge to moving forward in your life.

Thriving Means Letting Go of Your Story

I remember coming home from the Bahamas after being hit by the cement truck and telling everyone the story over and over again. I felt it was part of my healing. As mentioned in Chapter 2, a spiritual teacher/therapist lovingly confronted me and pointed out that I was too stuck in my story and highly recommended that it was time to let it go.

What is most important is what we can learn from our stories. These 13 Keys to Re-Empowerment were birthed as a result of that powerful encounter.

On your journey to becoming a thriver, there comes a point at which you have to let go of your story. You will know you're getting close to that point when you become bored telling the story one more time, and everybody around you is bored. In the beginning of your journey, your story serves you. Telling your story at that time is healthy, because it helps you process what happened. However, recognize the point at which it becomes unhealthy, and make an intention to make the shift and begin telling a new story so you can move forward.

Finding a New Normal

While many brain injury survivors say, *I want my old life back*, our life has become different. We can make an intention to embrace the differences as part of our journey and look for that new normal. Those of us with a brain injury are never ever going to be the same as we were prior to our injuries. Once we embrace that and find the new normal, we can have a wonderful life. We can continue to work on and improve our situation by acknowledging the small steps and small improvements. Every step from step A to B to C to D is a step in the right direction. Even when we experience a momentary memory loss, such as forgetting that a document we are looking for was left on the printer, we can stop and say, *Okay, I just had a moment*. We do not have to beat ourselves up as it is important to acknowledge that we are doing the best we can each moment, each day. It is important to change our mindset as we move back out into the world, learning to accept and take care of ourselves.

When I work, I work hard and put much time, effort, and energy into anything and everything I do. I have learned to work when my brain functions; there are times when it just does not function well. I've also learned that I need to plan time off so that I have the energy to work hard when needed. When I present a keynote speech, teach a workshop, design a training class, coach several clients per day, or facilitate a Survivor Series, I consciously do not plan anything else afterward except to have a little fun and rest. I know my reserves have been used up and that leads to cognitive fatigue. When preparing for these sessions, I'm jazzed; my adrenaline is surging and everything in me is operating at full steam. It takes longer to recover than it does for individuals without a brain injury, because a brain without an injury has more reserves. I am conscious and mindful of this and plan my life to successfully compensate.

When I introduce myself to people, I sometimes say that I have a brain injury, however I do not define myself as a brain-injured person. My intention is to be authentic, credible, and relatable. When I stand up in front of an audience of people with brain injuries, I begin with, "My name is Joanne Cohen, and I am a brain injury survivor or shall I say, thriver!" I say that to provide a connection and context as a person with multiple brain injuries. These injuries are frustrating at times, yet I have learned to embrace the limitations and recognize when they are frustrating me, usually when I am pushing myself too hard. I've learned to recognize the signs and accept my new normal.

Setting Boundaries

When I was a corporate executive, I had several incidents that were quite embarrassing. Part of living your life to the fullest is realizing when the fullest is full and knowing when to set boundaries for yourself. I crossed my own boundaries trying to keep commitments, because I always wanted and continue to want to be honorable and professional. I honored a commitment and learned a valuable painful lesson in the process. The boundaries I have learned to set include listening to my body, resting when I need to rest, giving my brain a break when I find myself losing things and forgetting things, and planning my calendar accordingly.

Later when I was working as a consultant, I was describing one of these painful incidents to my optometrist, Dr. Lynn Hellerstein. She described to me what was happening: I was experiencing brain freezes.

To explain what happens during a brain freeze, I'll share the following story:

I had made a commitment to my major and favorite client to fly to Miami to facilitate an off-site retreat with her executive leadership team. The session occurred after I had been rear-ended for a third time (more about this in Chapter 5), and after my cognitive therapist, Dr. Mary Ann Keatley, highly recommended I take three months off. I was in the acute brain injury stage after my three car accidents. She felt I was overdoing it, and my brain needed time to heal.

I responded, "That would be great, but I do not have time to take time off." I wanted to honor the commitment I made to my client and did not want to disappoint her. Not only was the work my bread-and-butter, I also loved working with the executives and especially this particular team. Against my doctor's advice, and against what my gut was screaming at me, I went to Miami to facilitate the two-day session.

The first day went well, and I met the expectations of my client and her team. After a long day, the team went out to dinner, and I joined them. In retrospect, this was not a good decision on my part. Looking back, it would have been best for my tired brain to go back to the hotel room, order in room service and rest, rather than eat a big meal, sip on some wonderful wine, and converse with folks. It was all fun, but it took additional cognitive energy.

We began the second day of the workshop, and I was more than exhausted. What I did not know then, but know now, is that my reserves were used up. I am typically able to rise to the occasion. However, with an acute brain injury, I rose as much as I was able to, but it just was not good enough for me or for my client. The morning of the second day, my gut intuition told me to recommend we put the session on hold for another time, as they were tired, and I was tired from the prior long day. However, I did not pay attention to my intuition. I bombed during my presentation. I usually set up a session so that everyone knows what to expect and why we're doing what we are doing. Instead, I jumped into the session on Emotional Intelligence, had pushback from one of the executives, had a brain freeze and totally forgot what I was saying. I did not handle the situation in my normal Joanne Cohen style. I did not feel like myself and disappointed everyone, including myself. I was there in body but not in mind. It was the most uncomfortable feeling when my brain shut down and I was unable to function cognitively. Since this is an invisible disability, no one knew or understood why I wasn't the consummate consultant they had grown accustomed to working with over the years. And I did not understand what was happening to me at the time. I was literally in survival mode. The meeting ended early and everyone left.

I was devastated and while flying home, wrote my raw feelings of anguish on a napkin. I felt like a failure, being the recovering perfectionist that I am. That was a very dark moment for me. I did not listen to my doctor's advice. I went because I did not want to let down the client, and I ended up failing both the client and me. I have learned that I am highly functioning until I am not. I used up my reserves, going over the reserve line without even knowing it. I will not make that mistake again—lesson learned.

My track record with that client up until this event was excellent. I had built credibility, trust, and respect with her and while she expressed her disappointment and gave me honest feedback, she kept me on as a consultant for her organization. I owned what happened (without ever using my brain injury as an excuse even though it was my reality) and apologized. I am proud to say that today I function much better. I am still consulting and accept engagements with this company, and we are continuing our relationship that will hopefully go on for many more years. It took me years to forgive myself for that experience in Miami.

A New and Different You

Live your life to the fullest as a new and different you. Embrace the new and different version of yourself, and live in the present, one moment at a time. The past is gone, and the future can be brighter even though it may be different than what you thought it was going to be. The brain you once had is gone. The brain you have now is the brain you have, and you can make improvements using various therapies. Mourn the loss of who you were with the intention of accepting the new and different you. Accepting the new mindset will enable you to live your life to the fullest. There are so many experts on this subject and so much work you can do to become better and thrive. Arthur Ashe said, "Start where you are. Use what you have. Do what you can."

That's Not the Truth About Me

When negativity is thrown your way, I have found the expression, *that's not the truth about me* to be helpful. When the physician assistant told me that I would not be able to walk or I would walk with a limp the rest of my life, and that this was as good as it gets, I could honestly say, *that's not the truth about me.* I continued to work diligently with my physical therapist for a year to prove them wrong, utilizing my inner strength and knowing this would not be my truth.

There are so many experts in the brain injury field who can support us to become better and work toward thriving in our life. You do not have to accept anybody telling you it's as bad as they say it is. Think of other survivors who were told they would never walk or talk again. They overcame their challenges because something bigger was driving them.

Key 2 – Focus on the *Ability* Not the *Dis*ability

When I write *dis*ability, I write *dis* very small and *ability* very big: dis*ability*. This is the difference between looking at the glass half empty, dis, and half full, *ability*. It is not my intention to deny having a disability, rather the intention is to focus on what can be done and what is needed for a better life.

Here is an example of when I was in *dis*ability mode: There are days when I thought, *Did I wash my hair? Did I put the conditioner on?* I had to compensate for this lapse in short-term memory by coming up with a solution I would remember, such as turning the shampoo and conditioner one way when it has been used and another way when it has not been used.

This might not sound like a big deal; however, I've been known to wash my hair several times because I immediately forgot if I did this or not—I had the cleanest hair in town! The point is, it feels disconcerting to not remember something that was so second nature to me prior to the accidents.

Years ago, I was in dis*ability* mode. I organized a Ropes Training for a cable company and the executive I worked with was very competitive. He had his team tackling big challenges so this was the perfect training event for this team. The challenge was to climb a telephone pole that looked about 80 feet high. It had rungs to climb up, and everyone wore a climbing harness and a helmet. When each person scaled the pole and got to the top, they jumped and grabbed a hanging trapeze and swung while the climbing harness kept them safe and out of harm's way. The CEO went up first and modeled the way for his team. Everyone clapped and screamed happily. One by one, each person climbed up and jumped. I watched in terror.

Knowing I had real issues with my injured neck, I thought, *Oh my goodness, how am I going to do this?!* I really do not have much neck and upper-body strength.

We all have inner strength, and it is important to tap into that inner strength and do the very best we can, and at the same time, know if we have real limitations and what they are. I am not a limitation person, nor do I focus on my limitations. With that being said, if something is going to hurt my neck causing me to have headaches for a week, I might choose not to do it.

I wasn't at the training for competitive reasons. I knew I would not be able to climb to the top of the pole. I tapped into my inner strength and started climbing. By the third rung, I was in agony from lifting myself from one rung to the next, putting pressure on my injured neck. That was as good as it was going to get for me. Everyone else got to the top and jumped, and I got up as high as I could. Surprising to me, the team still cheered me on, acknowledging what I *did* accomplish.

As I climbed down, I told myself to be happy because I made every effort to do my best and did not avoid the exercise or quit. It was a great lesson. I would love to have been able to climb to the top and jump like everyone else, and the truth was, I couldn't. I did my best because I focused on what I could do, not what I could not do. I focused on my *ability*, not my *dis*ability. I did part of it, and that was a win for me. I did not feel like I failed; I felt like I was very successful because I made an effort. The others knew I had issues and made an attempt to do this exercise anyway. I pushed past my fear. When I got to a certain pain point, I knew it was time to stop to avoid injuring myself further and ending up at the chiropractor for weeks. However, I did not just give in, pull the I'm-a-disabled-person card, and say, *I can't do this.* I did what I could, even if it was small. Celebrate those accomplishments in tiny increments with a can do attitude using positive thinking.

It is important for all of us to focus on what we can do, celebrate the small improvements and have as positive an attitude as possible. That does not mean we will not have bad days when we have been so cognitively fatigued that we cannot think. Personally, I just make every effort to regroup, recommit, and work hard to be the best possible version of myself, one day at a time. It helps tremendously to acknowledge our efforts, and not judge ourselves for things we used to be good at and can no longer do, or do not do as well as we did in the past. Just embrace where you are, who you are, and where you are at with as much glass-half-full perspective as you can. Keep moving from point A to point B to point C, however, do not discount that the depression, chronic pain, migraines, and a myriad of other things are real for people with a TBI. We're fortunate to live in an age when there are so many therapists and other professionals who do understand the brain injury community and can lend their support.

The most meaningful quote that has guided me throughout my life, especially throughout this journey with a brain injury, comes from a plaque that hangs in my office:

> God grant me the SERENITY
> To accept the things I cannot change,
> The COURAGE to change the things I can
> And WISDOM to know the difference.

I surely said the serenity prayer to myself as I looked up at that daunting 80-foot pole. For years I have found comfort and inspiration in these words. I keep a plaque with the inscription hanging in my office to this day. You may wish to select inspirational poems and quotes to support you and your life journey.

Key 3 – Acknowledge the Small Steps

A neuropsychologist and keynote speaker at a conference I once attended said, "Progress does not have a time stamp on it." Sometimes we think we should be better right now, yet we are a work in progress and must apply compensation strategies each step of the way. When we acknowledge the small steps, we can do so with an attitude of gratitude. In other words, appreciate any small recovery step that is in the right direction. For 27-plus years I have been moving from step to step and doing the very best I could in each moment. I have worked with many professionals who have been supportive and helpful, one step at a time: cognitive therapy, vision therapy, neuro-physical therapy, art therapy, music therapy, chiropractic, and so on.

In 2014, I was getting between four and five different therapies every week and finally said, "This is crazy! I'm burning out!" I was running from one to another not having enough time to get the homework done in between *and* working a full-time job. I had to take a step back and choose one or two and master them before moving on to another therapy—*small steps*!

I encourage you to acknowledge and be grateful for every positive thing that you do, no matter how small it is. Focus on acknowledging goals that you have set for yourself when you feel like I'm not where I was and I'm not where I want to be. Instead, acknowledge each small step because that's one step closer to being where you do want to be.

When I couldn't walk, my goal was to walk with crutches. When I met that goal, I wanted to walk with a cane. When I met that goal, I wanted to walk without a limp. When I met that goal, I wanted to walk part of the park pathway. When I accomplished that, I wanted to walk all the way around the park. Then I wanted to walk another park, which I did literally with small steps, focus, and intention. I felt such a sense of reward each step of the way.

It is the same with the brain. Break things into small increments and acknowledge every small step you achieve. Every night before you go to sleep, be grateful for every achievement. Grab a gratitude journal and write down everything you have accomplished that you are grateful for each day. When we focus on what we can't/don't do, we attract what we do not want. This can take us down a negative spiral and path. So, focus on what you *do* to attract what you want.

Embrace the positivity and the light about the greatness of something you accomplished. For instance, rather than thinking something is too small and no big deal, shift your thinking to, *it is a big deal.* It's a big deal if you didn't remember something and then it pops into your mind. Acknowledge that you remembered it. This is the glass half full rather than half empty philosophy, how you choose to frame your situation, and what your intentions are each and every day.

Key 4 – Be Your Own Advocate and Be Resourceful

Someone who attended our Survivor Series workshop once said to me, "Maybe *you* can be your own advocate, but I don't have it in me to be my own advocate." If that's true for you, then find someone who *will* advocate for you.

The following story shows what you can accomplish by being your own advocate, being resourceful, and working diligently. In 1980, prior to any brain injuries, I received a master's degree in speech communication from the University of Denver and earned all As and one B. Life was good! After my brain injury, I was anxious in crowds, had issues focusing and concentrating, and I was forgetful. I was in overload just like a computer that keeps shutting down. I was moody and frustrated and could not do the simple things I was able to do before the injury, such as balancing my bank accounts.

In 2010, I joined the training team at Denver Options (which later became Rocky Mountain Human Services) and worked with brain injury survivors. I went through the Academy of Certified Brain Injury Specialists (ACBIS) certification program sponsored by the Brain Injury Association of America (BIAA). This would be a meaningful credential in my role, and I would learn more about brain injury. An 80 percent is required to pass the challenging CBIS exam. I took the test, studied the way I had successfully studied in the past, and partnered with a colleague who was my CBIS Coach. After all that time, effort, and energy, I only received a 70 percent.

I failed the exam and was absolutely devastated.

BIAA allows everyone to take the exam twice, so I decided to take the test again, thinking, *You can't keep a good woman down. I'm going to pass that test!* The way I studied through graduate school had not worked with this exam. I knew I needed help and needed to be resourceful. I made an appointment to see Dr. Mary Ann Keatley, an exemplary, well known, and effective cognitive therapist who co-wrote the book *Understanding Mild Traumatic Brain Injury* (MTBI) with Laura Whittemore, former Executive Director for the Brain Injury Hope Foundation. I worked with

Dr. Keatley for six months, focusing on how to take tests, actually taking practice tests, and learning to study a different way so I could pass the test the second time around. I discovered that I needed to work on my speed of processing, my short-term memory, and some other areas in which I had tested below the mean (being compared to others who had a master's degree at my age) during cognitive testing.

I also knew that I needed to be my own advocate. Prior to taking the test I contacted the BIAA, which administers the exam, and asked for specific accommodations. The first time I took the exam, it was on the computer. I asked to take a written exam with a pencil and paper, because I learned a technique from Dr. Keatley involving underlining and circling information. I also asked to take the exam in a quiet room by myself. The first time I took the exam, I was in a cubicle in a room with other people, and it was too noisy. I wasn't able to fully concentrate. I asked for accommodations and, with the help of my boss, now my business partner, they agreed. This time I scored a 94 percent! By working hard, being resourceful, and being my own advocate, I was able to succeed in becoming a Certified Brain Injury Specialist (CBIS), a proud moment in my life and career.

I've heard it said that people with a brain injury cannot get better after 18 months. In my experience, that is not true. My accident was in 1992, and I received my certification 19 years later. My score shows that we can get better if we position ourselves to work with the right people who truly know how to help us, and we are willing to put in the extra effort. Bottom line: be your own advocate and find those great people who will accept and support you. And, do not believe or buy into everything you are told. Let the information motivate you to find professionals who will believe in you, have a treatment that *can* help you, and work like heck to move the needle and make small steps in the right direction. Embrace the words, "God, give us grace to accept with serenity the things that cannot be changed, courage to change the things which should be changed, and the wisdom to distinguish the one from the other."

Take responsibility for your healing, or find an advocate, whether a professional, a friend, a caregiver, a colleague, a significant other/partner, or a family member. It is important to partner and surround yourself with people who truly love and support you.

Some examples of advocating:

You advocate for yourself when you sign up for Supplemental Security Income (SSI) and Social Security Disability Income (SSDI).

You become your own advocate when you find someone to support you when you're having a challenging brain day. Others can help you get to a Survivor Series/other BI training events or fill out forms or manage your checkbook. After my injury, my friends, my woman's group, my Geneva Group (which is my spiritual family)—people who love and care about me, reached out and were very supportive.

Seek out events sponsored by the brain injury community and network with other BI survivors and professionals who understand your injury and challenges.

Seek out professionals who understand brain injury

and have a treatment plan that can support you and your recovery process.

One of my advocates is a neighbor, Lois Florkey, who, after my partner passed away, took on the role of office organizer, and believe me, *that* was a challenge! John Ramiraz, a wonderful friend for many years, has his own to do list and comes over to help me with household activities that require heavy lifting, sweeping the garage, cleaning the grill, and other activities that would exacerbate my body issues. I play to my strengths and bring in others who play to their strengths to support me.

When you find an organizer, be sure he or she organizes in a way that helps you the way your brain thinks, not the way their brain thinks. Share with him or her what organizational system works for you. If you do not know, you can co-create a system together. My neighbor learned more about brain injury through me. She now knows the questions to ask so that we file or organize things that work for my brain. She knows to ask, "This is what I would do—will that work for you?" I am so appreciative to have Lois and John as advocates and friends on my support team.

Your partner, significant other, or spouse can also be your advocate. Roni came into my life in 1995, post brain injury. We cared for each other and understood each other's strengths. It was not a big deal if I'd say, "I've got this presentation. Here are my notes. Can you put them in the right format? Then I can take it from there."

I was walking into a neighborhood store and saw a woman and her husband getting ready to ride their recumbent bikes. I am unable to ride a regular bike as it hurts my neck. I asked the woman if she liked her recumbent bike and if she would recommend it. She introduced herself as Karen and responded, "Oh yes, I'm a brain injury survivor." She opened up right away, telling me about her brain injuries, how this bike is different from a regular bike, and discussed her balance and other BI-related issues. A light bulb went off for me. I let her know that we were putting together a Survivor Series panel in 2018, and I asked her if she would like to be on the panel of BI survivors. She in turn invited me to speak at her church about brain injury. Karen was able to be her own advocate in selecting the right bike for herself and I was resourceful in seeing an opportunity to invite Karen to share her experiences with the brain injury community at the Survivor Series.

Key 5 – Consider Medical and Complementary Therapies

As you consider medical and complementary therapies, trust the process, and do the work. I recommend working with the traditional medical community in addition to selecting the therapies that complement them.

There are so many healing options and it may be challenging to know where to begin. Every brain injury is unique, so tailor who and what you might choose for your own particular needs. If you are not sure, select a BI professional who can help you navigate your way through all your choices and options to select what will be best for you in your own unique situation.

I was fortunate enough to receive $2,000 in 2011 from the Colorado Traumatic Brain Injury Trust Fund that I used to work with therapists who specialize in traditional and complementary modalities. There are so many incredible professionals in the field that it actually becomes challenging to decide where to focus. When we assemble brain injury teams and panels, it is exciting to have so many choices of professionals who show up lovingly and willingly, giving their time to embrace the community they serve and frequently offering discounts or a free initial exam.

For instance, on one panel for brain injury treatment therapies, we included Dr. John Hughes, who spoke about hyperbaric oxygen therapy; Dr. Robert Gardner, an audiologist, who talked about vertigo and tinnitus; Beth Fishman McCaffrey from Hellerstein & Brennan Vision Center who discussed vision therapy; and Nancy Bonifer, a neuro-physical therapist, who shared information about her understanding of how to work with a BI client when giving physical therapy assignments. Neuro-chiropractors Dr. Shawn VanWinkle and Dr. Shane Steadman, and a retired trauma-release therapist, Marilyn Coonelly, also shared their insights about how they have and are helping clients with brain injuries using their methodology.

Other therapies include cognitive therapy, rehabilitative Qigong and Tai Chi, Eye Movement Desensitization and Reprocessing (EMDR), adaptive yoga, Integrated Listening System (a neuro-application of the Tomatis Method), psychotherapy, assistive technology tools, acupuncture, equine-assisted therapy, energy work, cranial cerebral therapy, cannabidiol (CBD) oil, essential oils, occupational therapy, sleep regulation, art therapy, music therapy, recreational therapy, NeurOptimal (a form of neurofeedback), Logosynthesis, and the importance of diet and nutrition, especially important for those of us with brain injuries. The list of exemplary practitioners and treatments goes on and on. The biggest challenge and frustration for many in our community is finding the funds to pay for these treatments. Some are covered by insurance, and some are private pay. Some people have limited funds and often no insurance at all. Lack of financial resources is a big issue in the brain injury community, and we are, unfortunately, an under-served community regarding funding resources.

A wellness approach is also recommended. According to Dr. Mary Ann Keatley, wellness is a three-pronged approach: body, mind, and spirit. You can enhance your physical wellness by paying attention to exercise, rest, diet, and fluids. Your diet might include more power foods, such as dark chocolate, blueberries, nuts, especially walnuts, oranges, and coffee beans. You can enhance your mental wellness by practicing meditation, guided imagery, and relaxation techniques. You can enhance your spiritual wellness by focusing on prayer, forgiveness, spending time in nature, giving up control, having an attitude of gratitude, understanding the power of intention, and living in the now to achieve future goals. (To remind yourself to live in the moment, consider a now watch.) Discover what will work best for you in your journey through brain injury.

Although having so many complementary therapies to choose from is exciting, and as I mentioned previously, I found myself becoming exhausted going through so many therapies at the same time. It became impossible to do the homework, because all I was doing was running from one therapy to another, a common mistake made by many of us because we are so determined to feel, to be, and to get better. I discussed this with Dr. Keatley, who had already suggested that I slow down. We decided that I should focus only on vision therapy, therapies that enhance the connection between my eyes and my brain, and chiropractic treatments for the chronic body pain. She believed cognitive therapy would work better once the vision issues were handled. I reset my intention to do everything in moderation.

If you are unable to figure out what to do, go to a professional who can help you, one who is not self-serving. Look for someone who is working with BI clients for the right reasons—who sincerely wants to help you and has a track record of getting results. Work with people who do it from the heart and have a passion for their work, versus the people who are not in the field for the right reasons, who only care about the money and suck off the misfortune of others' hardships. Work with professionals who you feel comfortable with and do not judge you. I like to find out why they got into their line of work, what motivates them and what keeps them up at night. The intention of the practitioner is important to me, as Marsha Sinetar's book title states, *Do What You Love The Money Will Follow.*

As you shift through traditional and nontraditional therapies, select what works for you. For me, it was cognitive therapy, massage therapy, vision therapy, chiropractic, and neuro-physical therapy care. I added an attorney to my team. With three accidents in 2014, the paperwork was so overwhelming, I chose to not do this on my own and instead retain an attorney. I'll share more about this in Chapter 6.

To manage your resources and fatigue, pay attention to diet and exercise, get enough sleep, take naps, and plan for energy-consuming activities. For example, after I give a presentation, I might have a two-hour massage, or take a hot bath and light a candle to relax to take care of myself.

Know when you are at your best and plan your day accordingly. For instance, if you're at your best in the morning, plan to schedule meetings at that time. Identify and recognize when you get overwhelmed. Get treatment if you need it. Consider support therapy, Employee Assistance Programs (EAPs) and/or grief counseling. You may experience grief over the loss of who you were and who you are now.

Some people need medication management; others need job accommodations.

The reason I love providing the Survivor Series is because in our BI community people tend to isolate themselves, and social isolation is not always good for healing the mind and spirit. The Survivor Series helps participants interact with each other. You might look fine to others; however that does not mean it is how you really feel. Social interaction takes effort. Sometimes you are comfortable with it and other times you may not be. It is important to develop your social skills and get out in the world. It is important to honor those times when you need to isolate yourself. It is equally important to honor those times when you feel like kicking yourself out the door because it's not healthy to totally isolate yourself. Get involved. Attend support groups. Work. Volunteer. Focus on what's working. You'll get a greater sense of empowerment, self-identity, and self-esteem. You'll establish a feeling of purpose. You'll develop new skills and learn new things. That's empowerment.

Key 6 – Develop a Support Team and Advocacy Network

Developing a support team and advocacy network will help you *thrive!*

Put together your dream team. Getting well means taking action. Network to find others who are brain injury survivors, so you do not feel so alone. We build community and a sense of belongingness with the Brain Injury Hope Foundation's Survivor Series. Everyone is at a different stage in their journey. It helps to find people with similar issues so you will not feel so alone.

As you actively find those who will join your support team, look for professionals who encourage you, who understand you, and who do not discount your capabilities and progress. Seek those who encourage and reinforce your small steps and progress.

One client said to me, "Yeah, they told me to go see a psychiatrist because it's all in my head—no pun intended." Well, it's all in your brain, but it's not all in your mind. Psychotherapy can help you deal with some of the psychological ramifications of your injury—and can be an important part of your healing in addition to what we discussed in Key 5. It is not a sign of weakness to seek out help. It is a sign of strength and courage.

I've had different dream teams over the years. After the three car accidents in 2014, my dream team was made up of neuro-PT, Nancy Bonifer; cognitive therapist, Mary Ann Keatley; chiropractor, Dr. Bill Borman; attorney, Rebecca Albano (who later joined the Brain Injury Hope Foundation board); vision therapist, Dr. Lynn Hellerstein; neurologist, Dr. Heidi Ray; and dietician, Kim Gollick. (People with brain injuries in the acute state might find that they gain weight—perhaps 30 to 40 pounds. I gained 30 pounds. I added a grief counselor, Rita Coalson, after losing my partner of 21 years to leukemia in 2016 (more about that in Chapter 7).

The hospice grief counselor was valuable because when a significant person passes, not only do you grieve that loss, you also grieve any loss you have experienced in the past. It brings up grief for the loss of your father, your mother, your aunts, your uncles, your dogs, and your cats, and anyone else you have lost.

I lost my partner while I was still healing from multiple brain injuries. When someone close to you dies, the grief produces symptoms like an acute brain injury. This was a very difficult time for me. I got through this with the help and support of everyone on my dream team. (See Chapter 7 to learn more about grief and grieving after a brain injury.)

As you assemble your dream team, keep in mind that it is important to do bodywork such as massage, chiropractic adjustments, reiki, and craniosacral therapy. If you can afford it and your body is able to receive this healing touch, it can be very beneficial. In fact, when I was cutting down on the number of therapies, I made sure to keep massage and chiropractic on my schedule. Again, find what works best for *you.*

Key 7 – Move out of the Closet and into the World

Some survivors are writing books, poetry, and speaking at conferences. I have done some of these things, and I find it very freeing. For me it has been rewarding to get up in front of an audience and say, "I'm Joanne, I'm a TBI survivor." After years of being in the closet, I chose to be open about my brain injury. I chose to write this book and speak publicly on panels and at conferences.

In my professional life, I worried about disclosing that I had a brain injury. Especially in an interview, I was afraid I wouldn't get the job because of it. If I did get the job, I was afraid I might get fired if I disclosed. This created a lot of stress.

Then I began to meet with friends who shared their own TBI experiences. I did not know they were injured. When they began sharing their experiences with me, it encouraged me to come out about my own TBI and this helped tremendously.

The truth will set you free. Fear is actually **F**alse **E**vidence that **A**ppears **R**eal. Disclosure is a gray area, not black and white. The jobs I thrived in were ones in which my bosses knew I was recovering from a TBI and provided the necessary accommodations such as teleworking and taking time off when necessary. See Chapter 4 for more information about managing a career with a brain injury.

Telling people about your brain injury can be very difficult. There are pros and cons to disclosure. Go with your gut instincts. Sometimes your mind can say one thing and your gut another. You want to feel safe, you want to trust, and you want to feel that you *can* trust. Ask yourself, *What's the worst that could happen if I tell my family, my friends, or my boss? Can I live with their reactions or responses?* Look at your fears. Are they false evidence that appears real or are they real fears and danger? You might be afraid you'll be fired. You might be afraid you'll be discounted, rejected, or judged. To disclose or not to disclose—that is the question, and the answer is a personal one for each and every one of us.

I've been hired, I've been fired, I've laughed, and I've cried. It is about moving out of the closet and into the world. You have to do it in a way that feels comfortable to you. I'm not saying to disclose to the world that you have a brain injury or multiple brain injuries—this is and will always be your choice and your story to tell. Choose to do what is right for you.

Key 8 – Ask for Help

It takes a courageous person to ask for help. Some people believe if they ask for help it will make them look weak. I firmly believe it shows strength to ask for help and to let people advocate for you. I have asked and continue to ask for help. There are things I can do and things I just cannot do. Many times, I hire people and other times people lend support out of the goodness of their hearts and I sometimes accept that. I ask people to gently remind me if I repeat myself. I ask people to send me emails about what we discussed so I will remember the information. It is okay to ask people to help you compensate for the things you are unable to do yourself or if you feel challenged.

In the beginning, I felt like no one was on my side and no one understood me. I felt discounted and shut down. Brain injury survivors commonly say, *No one gets me.* We are not crazy, lazy, stupid, or dumb. We're that person who says, *I'm not a brain-injured person; I'm a person with a brain injury.* Let people know how you need to be supported, no matter how difficult that becomes. And, if they know you need support and you do not know, consider accepting the support when offered.

Find people who understand people with brain injuries. Sometimes, we do not know when we need to ask for help. That's when our friends and advocates play an important role in our lives. Asking for help is an act of courage, and I have personally learned how to ask for and accept support. Most of the time, I pay for the help I ask for because I believe in the exchange of energy (in the form of money). I do not want to feel beholden. I never want to feel like I'm taking advantage of my friends or have them feel this way; at the same time, I have learned to accept their gift of time and help when appropriate. To give is to receive and to receive is to give—one of life's most valuable lessons.

Key 9 – Compensate, Compensate, COMPENSATE!

One way to compensate is to use the assistive devices available to you such as Siri and GPS. I was directionally impaired before my brain injuries and even more so after, so these assistive devices are extremely helpful.

One day, I was driving to see a movie with a friend. I had been to that theatre many times; however, on that occasion, I just could not remember how to get to that movie theatre. The more I couldn't find it, the more stressed I became. The more stressed I became, the more I couldn't find it. I called my friend from two blocks away and asked her for the address. I knew I was in the neighborhood. I put the address in my GPS and finally arrived, just in time for the movie to begin.

Another time, I drove to a conference in Colorado Springs and realized I forgot my TempurPedic neck pillow. I had brain fog, and I wasn't able to put a list together on what to pack. I cannot sleep on any other pillow; I would be in agony. I also forgot my purse and my cash.

Unbelievable, yet anyone with a brain injury could relate, right? This is how cognitive fatigue shows up for me. I know now that I have to be intentional and make a list for traveling to help me remember everything that is needed. I am now the proud owner of three neck pillows because that wasn't the first time I forgot my pillow! By using notes, I have avoided buying a fourth neck pillow.

I put keys in the same place every day, or I will not find them. As I mentioned before, when I wash and condition my hair, I turn each bottle the opposite way, so I know I have done this. I work with an organizer and use sticky notes to stay organized (even though my current organizer wants me to get rid of those sticky notes). These are just a few ways to compensate for challenges.

It has been said that the definition of insanity is doing the same thing over and over and expecting different results. If we do not come up with ways to compensate, we will get more stressed. Continue doing what works, discontinue doing what doesn't work. Look at ways that you can compensate. If you need help, work with your professionals, your advocates, your family members, your friends, and your caregivers.

As you learn to compensate, use the right language. Your subconscious does not understand the negative. For instance, rather than saying, *Don't forget to turn off the water*, say, *Remember to turn off the water.* Or even better, say to your partner or spouse, *Please help me remember to turn off the water.* I've flooded my basement more than once and now keep this advice in mind.

What ways do you compensate for your challenges?

Key 10 – Be Patient with Others Who Don't Understand

Learn to deal compassionately with the human side of yourself, your family, your friends, your colleagues, and medical professionals. This can be quite challenging when one feels disempowered by others and takes a great deal of patience.

Voice your needs. One morning, my friend John was planning to come over and help me clean my basement, but I wasn't up to it. I called him and said, "Can we please renegotiate this? I really want to clean the basement, but I am exhausted and have a very important presentation tomorrow. I would like to reschedule for a week from Friday." He was fine with it. He understood. I gave him a gift of time, and he gave me a gift of time. It is okay to ask people to accommodate your needs as long as you are respectful of them and of their time.

Learning about the Limited Capacity Model was an important gift. This model gives us a way to explain our cognitive fatigue to others. When I could not find my way to the movie, I said to my friend, "I'm so sorry. I just couldn't connect. I am so cognitively fatigued." He said to me, "I get fatigued, too." These types of statements are common and meant to be supportive. However, while it may be unintentional, the person with a brain injury can feel discounted and what they have expressed is not being taken seriously.

Using the Limited Capacity Model[2], I was able to explain to him that the brain is like a pie. A healthy brain injury can be under cognitive, physical, and emotional stress and use a little less than half of the pie to deal with that stress. This brain still has the other half of the pie in reserve. The person with a healthy brain can bounce back quickly from challenging circumstances. Everyone is different, and my brain injury causes me to use more than three-quarters of my brain pie to function on a day-to-day basis. That means that I have very little pie left to deal with other things and therefore have fewer reserves.

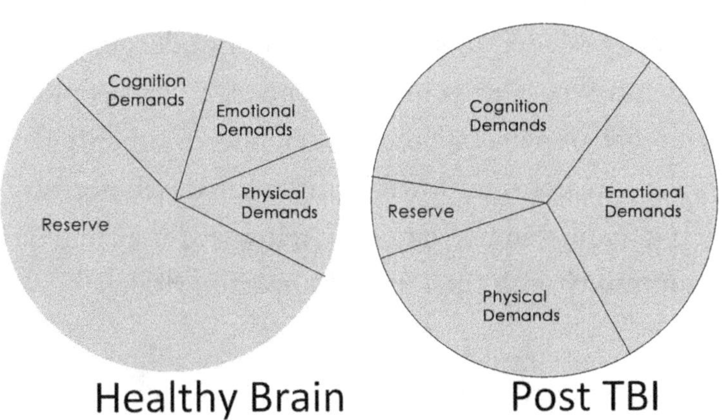

Healthy Brain   Post TBI

Less Reserve = More Demand

"Mary Lou Acimovic, Limited Capacity Model"

Mary Lou Acimovic, MA, CCC-SP, wrote about the Limited Capacity Model in *Mild Traumatic Brain Injury: The Guidebook*. This model gives us the words to explain how having a TBI changes one's cognitive, physical, and emotional energy level and describes the differences between a healthy brain and a post-TBI brain. This model helps to explain that you are not playing the victim or making things up; you are taking steps to care for yourself by preserving energy or resting after you have overextended yourself. Be patient with yourself and with others. This model helps people understand brain injury limitations and perhaps, as others are introduced to this model, they will become more patient and understanding. Use the Limited Capacity Model to help others better understand you, your process, and your experience. As the people in your life understand the model, the comments that make you feel shut down or dishonored will decrease. A big thank you to Mary Lou Acimovic for gifting our community with the Limited Capacity Model.

Years ago, the owner and main facilitator of a fabulous leadership development workshop became frustrated with me because I needed to use notes to co-facilitate the workshop with her. She did not need or use notes and expected all contractors to do the same. It was a requirement for the job. There is and was no way, no how, in this lifetime, that I can learn and/or facilitate without taking and using notes. Even when I disclosed my brain injury, she was not happy with me using notes. I know this frustrated my colleague and impacted our working relationship. This can be challenging for those of us with this invisible disability—it just does not make sense to some people.

When I went from wheelchair to crutches to one crutch to a cane, my disability was visible. Walking and looking as I do now, it became invisible. Somebody said, "Be kind, for everyone you meet is fighting a hard battle." I thought that was meaningful.

You can disclose your injury or keep quiet about it. If you do disclose your injury, the intent of that disclosure is to inform and create a better understanding of your situation and is not meant to be used as an excuse or to characterize yourself as a victim. And if you disclose, be prepared to ask yourself, *What is the worst that can happen if I do disclose it?*

Key 11 – Know that Helping Others IS Helping Yourself

The eleventh key is to know that helping others *is* helping yourself.

I believe in giving to give, not giving to get. Even though it may not be your intention, you end up getting when you do give. In 2010, while working in the corporate world, I was invited to do a Survivor Series for CTAT at Denver Options in Denver, Colorado because one of my colleagues had to cancel due to the effects of cancer treatments. By the end of that presentation I thought, for the first time, that I was a part of a community. I felt like I did not have to be perfect. I could forget what I lost. I could experience a brain freeze and just say, *Oh! I don't know where I was, where I am, or where I'm going.* The audience and I would have a good laugh! People would laugh *with* each other, not *at* each other. That day, I understood at a deep level that helping others is helping yourself. I still like the intention of helping others without the expectation of receiving anything in return. Helping others is being of service and being there for others.

This reminds me of a story that illustrates how helping others helps yourself. A colleague's wife, who was very quiet and nice, was going through a life challenge. We did not know each other well. On a day when she was not feeling as positive as usual, she showed up in my hospital with a small balloon and said, "Hi!" As she waved that balloon, I remember sitting up as straight as I could while still in painful traction. Both of our hearts opened. I was so touched that this woman came to see me, and it made both of us feel so much better in that moment. Out of her feelings of ups and downs, she said, "I'm not going to stay at home today. I'm going to do something to help someone else today." I was just an acquaintance, but she made a decision to go to the hospital and visit me and that changed both of our lives for the better. We became very close friends and are friends to this day. We became neighbors for a few years. We went through mourning, ups and downs, and the grief process together, each for different reasons. I will always value and appreciate this friendship that began while I was in the hospital in 1992.

When my friend, Linda Fankboner, came to visit me in the hospital and made the chocolate and champagne party for me, I know how happy she felt creating this experience. I also felt so much better in those moments of pain to do something fun with such a caring and considerate friend. We speak about it to this day!

After I was released from the hospital and in the next stage of recovery at home, Linda and I discussed going to Boulder, Colorado to hear Stephen Levine discuss his perspective regarding death and dying. I was still in a wheelchair. My physical therapist taught Linda how to get me in and out of the wheelchair and how to fold the wheelchair and get it into the car. That night, Linda picked me up and we drove to Boulder. We had the best seats in town because I was in that wheelchair! Again, I am so appreciative of the outpouring of support from Linda and other friends that reached out to me at one of the most challenging times in my life. It made me feel cared for and loved. I believe these friends and colleagues felt good, too, knowing they made such a positive difference in my life. Helping each other *is* helping yourself. We forged an incredible bond and built strong relationships.

People did things for me, and that is what I have done ever since, meeting and connecting with survivors and paying it forward. With the help of resources and grants, the Brain Injury Hope Foundation hosts the Survivor Series, and I organize and facilitate most of the sessions. Before this opportunity, I was "working for a dying" as Joe Dominguez wrote in *Your Money or Your Life* instead of "working for a living." I thought I would be more at peace and more comfortable working full-time in corporations, but that was not the case. Since leaving the corporate world and working as a consultant in my own business, I have been able to pay it forward more often. Again, helping others *is* helping yourself!

Key 12 – Choose Your Journey, Your Life: Everything Happens for a Reason

The twelfth key is to choose your journey, your life: Everything happens for a reason. When you are ready, ask yourself, what was the reason for my injury and what will I do as a result of what happened to me?

For me, the accidents happened for more than one reason. Throughout the years, looking through my rearview mirror, I came to understand what those reasons are—not only surviving this journey, but thriving. In 2014, I had a major setback, (disclosed in Chapter 5) and had to go back into a number of therapies with the goal to thrive again and reach my next new normal. My commitment is to continuous quality improvement, and I will always commit to raising my own bar.

I asked myself, *What am I going to do to help others now that I've arrived home?* I arrived home as a survivor and a thriver by working with CTAT, LLC and the Brain Injury Hope Foundation, my two passions.

Another brain injury survivor, Jeffrey Therrien, who started a company called Purpose Writers, wrote, "The time has come to learn to fall in love with the punches of life and how to handle them. This is quite the realization and that alone is huge."

In one of his articles, he wrote:[3]

Personally, I've spent the last five years or so in the whitewater rapids. I've been tossed around, playing survival, enjoying some moments, regretting the occasional mistake, getting off course, back on course and off course again, simply hoping and praying for that moment when the water is still once more. That peaceful spot in the river where we can adjust our posture, realign ourselves with our true circumstance and wisely choose our path. This stillness, this ability to take a quick look at the big picture is what many of us with a troubled brain live without. This leads us to the simple question. What happens to those who are in the midst of their adventure? Tossed off the canoe and forced in a world that is chaotic inside and out when they have not a penny saved and are living paycheck to paycheck in order to survive in the first place? Waking up as a new person in a new world, losing health insurance, in addition to losing their income? That is the question that inspired the letter; what does one do? I offer this example to put things in perspective.

And then he writes, "Let us step into the shoes of a TBI survivor for a moment." One survivor shared, "Things work out the best for those who make the best out of how things work out." Winnie the Pooh says, "Promise you'll always remember you're braver than you believe and stronger than you seem in spite of what you think." There is a quote on a T-shirt I saw that says, I am therefore I matter. Again, write down the quotes and poems that inspire you to help you as you move through. It is a great exercise for brain injury survivors and inspirational too.

Yes, this *is* the journey!

Key 13 – Use Resiliency to Survive and Thrive

Resiliency is a mindset, an intention, a focus, and a belief that you *can* get up and move beyond. An example is putting your dream team together to figure out what you can do and then choosing to do it and selecting the right people to be on your team. This is instrumental to supporting a mindset of resiliency with the goal to move from surviving to thriving.

Like 2014, 2015 was a challenging year, to say the least. I broke my wrist and then I broke my big toe. My entire team, my boss, and I had our positions eliminated. This had been the best job I ever had, so my boss and I formed a new business, and she has been my business partner going on five years. My life partner, Roni, had her job eliminated, too, and then we lost our beloved cat, Moe. The next year, on December 13, 2016, I lost my partner of 21 years to leukemia. Through each one of these losses, resiliency played a role in being able to get hit, get up, and move beyond. There was pain and grief to experience and embrace. I worked with a grief counselor after the death of my beloved. Doing this grief work (see Chapter 7) was the best decision I made and truly helped me get up. Resiliency!

We go through so much grief because of our brain injury and because we are forced to change how we live our lives. Many of us have done that over and over again. Getting hit, getting up, getting hit, getting up… losing my partner was a major hit. I discovered with my grief therapist that grief put me back in a state of acute brain injury. It was exhausting, ugly, and messy. The only way out was to go through the process. In the process of getting re-empowered while adjusting to a new way of life, I've learned a lot about myself. Yes, the key to moving from surviving to thriving is to make it an intention to be resilient.

Two roads diverged in a wood, and I—
I took the one less traveled by,
And that has made all the difference.

Robert Frost

Chapter 4
Maintaining a Career

My career was and still is very important to me and is in alignment with my purpose: To add value, make a difference, and bring humanity into whatever I do. I started out teaching high school English, Speech, and Drama in Elmira, New York. After receiving a master's degree from the University of Denver in 1979, I settled in Colorado and ventured into the corporate world, working my way up the chain from a Training Coordinator to Training Supervisor, Manager, and Director positions. The best fit for me were positions where I could work in individual contributor roles. In addition to the corporate arena, I have worked in the non-profit sector, for consulting firms, self-employment, and in roles as an internal and as an external consultant. I have owned my own business twice: once as a sole proprietor and in my current business as a limited liability company with my business partner (and former boss), Gayann Brandenburg.

At the time I was hit by the cement truck, I was self-employed and had working relationships with an outplacement firm and a local Employee Assistance Program (EAP). I kept my business going for a while, as well as working as a consultant with the outplacement firm on a contract basis. The EAP relationship ended while I was still in recovery from this horrific accident. I was making every effort to get back into my work life, and even collaborated with a consultant to design a beautiful brochure for Joanne Cohen Associates. I found myself giving the brochure to friends and not marketing to the right people or putting myself out there. At the time, I did not realize I had a closed-head brain injury; however, I knew something wasn't quite right. It was shortly afterwards that I learned about the TBI.

I have an outstanding resume and curriculum vitae; however, I found I had to work twice as hard and work longer hours to be as productive as I had been before the accident. It took a toll on me, causing undo stress, discomfort, and cognitive fatigue that would not end. At the time, I did not know that my decisions to accept bigger and bigger job opportunities were not the best decisions for me. I followed a path as if I were someone without a brain injury. I was responding as if I was who I used to be prior to the accidents and not who I was in my new normal condition.

The Good, Bad, Ugly, and Great

I decided to follow a good friend's advice to leave my business and apply for a corporate position because I did not know what I could and could not do anymore. I was awarded the job. This ended up being a *huge* job—a position as the West Region Training Manager for a cell phone company start-up. This was the biggest position of my career and my life! While there are successes that I am proud of to this day, I have to be honest and admit that this job was way too big for my cognitive capabilities resulting from an untreated brain injury. Today this makes me smile, but at the time, it was not funny when I was labeled *the sticky queen* because I had sticky notes all over my office in an effort to retain everything I needed to know and remember.

Another situation arose when my boss confronted me about the number of notes I was taking, as she said there was a perception that I was not listening. I did not know at the time I was struggling with speed-of-processing issues and compensating by taking notes on everything I heard as fast as I could, and then reading the notes. That *was* my form of listening. There was so much to learn quickly, and I was in overload all the time. While I did not disclose to her that I had a brain injury out of fear of getting fired, I did inform my boss that "this *is* the way I listen, and please do not ask me to not take notes again." Fortunately, she complied with my request.

A few years later, I worked for a fantastic boss, David Birks, in an individual contributor position and was very successful. We built trust with each other. I proved myself quickly, and it was easy to disclose my brain injury issues and what I needed from him to be successful. He was a great business partner and lent support and accommodations when needed. I loved working with him and at that company. However, we knew the company was looking to merge with or to be acquired by another company, and that the work I was doing in leadership development would probably be eliminated. So, I chose to leave the best job and boss I had ever had up until that time for another corporate job in a position managing people again. In this job, there were extremely high expectations in a culture that was not a fit for me or for my cognitive needs and functioning.

I moved from company to company, to larger and larger positions, making more and more money, and reached my goal of making six figures. There was a tremendous cost to me and to those who worked with me. I was hired and fired from some positions. I was hired and very successful in other positions. What made the difference for me was the environment, the type of boss I worked with and for, the team I was working with, and working in an individual contributor role versus a role as a manager with many direct reports. I finally understood that my brain injury was the real deal. I needed to work in a different environment with a different type of boss where accommodations could be made so I could enjoy success as well as take care of myself. This is the powerful formula for maintaining a career with a brain injury. I do not and have not defined myself by my brain injury. However, over time, I have learned that my brain injury is something to be acknowledged. Cognitive fatigue, brain fog, and brain freeze are the by-product of working too many long hours or working in an environment that is not a fit for my hidden/invisible disability.

After leaving that biggest job of my career in 2010, I decided to drop out of corporate America and join a non-profit organization, taking a 60 percent cut in pay. I was fortunate enough to work with and for a boss (my current business partner) who hired me knowing I had a brain injury. She understood brain injury without being judgmental, and she provided the accommodations I needed to succeed. I could telework on an as-needed basis, I could work shorter days and make up the time as needed, and I could take time off when needed. It was a winning formula, the perfect fit, and for that I am forever thankful. After five years, we were all laid off due to funding cuts. Gayann and I went into business together and formed **Coaching, Training and Transformation**, LLC—CTAT, LLC, and we each play to our strengths. We also became leaders on the board of directors for the Brain Injury

Hope Foundation (BIHF), a non-profit organization that provides emergency funds for mild to moderate TBI survivors in Colorado. We added the Survivor Series to what we offer. I am project manager for the series, which is funded by donations and grants, and facilitate many of the monthly sessions.

Lessons Learned

There are many lessons learned along the way; I hope these will be useful to you or someone you know with a brain injury or injuries:

- If you plan to return to work, be cognizant of your strengths and cognitive abilities. Select work that is a good fit for who you are today, not who you were prior to your brain injury.

- The environment and the people you work with are critical to your happiness, successes, and/or failures. Select wisely.

- Remember, an interview is a two-way street. You have an opportunity to select a boss, a team, and an environment that appreciates diversity and supports/accepts people with disabilities.

- To disclose or not to disclose—that is the question. I learned that my best successes were with bosses who knew I had a brain injury, were supportive, and happily provided accommodations.

- If you are fortunate enough to be able to accept doing what you love, life will unfold with more positivity.

- Turning a hobby into a profession can be a consideration as you figure out what's next. If you find a position that ends up not being a good fit, move on quickly rather than staying, suffering, and ending up either being asked to resign or getting fired.

- Perhaps you might want to consider putting the pieces together—getting a part-time job and doing some volunteer work while working on your recovery and attending healing appointments. Or perhaps selecting one piece and starting somewhere! For some of you, it may be something that will complement or enhance your Supplemental Security Income (SSI) or Social Security Disability Income (SSDI.)

- If you get testing and feedback from a doctor, therapist, etc., the results might say you are unable to work (they have to say this so you can qualify for benefits), and only you can make this decision.

- You may think about accepting a position/job that may not seem to be your perfect idea of what you want to do; however, this position can lead to another future position that is more desirable.

- Your recovery may be your full-time job for quite a while; let that be okay.

- For those of you who are unable to return to work or return to what you were doing prior to your TBI, explore all financial means and benefits that will help you pay the bills, focus on your recovery, and find what brings you joy as you create your life as the new you.

- Work with a coach to help you figure out what transferrable skills you have and what would be a good fit for you. A coach will also help you face any and all fears you have.

- You may not know what kinds of accommodations you will need when you first accept a job; however, over time, this will unfold. If you want accommodations, you will then need to disclose your TBI to human resources or your boss in order for the accommodations to be provided.

- If you cannot perform the duties with an accommodation, it may be time to look for something else that is a better fit, either within or outside the company. If you make that choice, it may be easier emotionally versus getting fired. Don't be afraid to acknowledge your limitations and reality.

- Self-employment became the best fit for me so I could control my environment, time, energy, who I work with (and choose to not work with), projects, the hours I work, etc. You will have to assess what works best for you.

- Isolation can be detrimental; find something that motivates you to get out of the house.

- Again, use the serenity prayer if it resonates with you, to help deal with any feelings and emotions that can get in the way of moving forward.

Don't Give Up!

The wisdom and the clarity I am able to share with you is a result of me looking into a rearview mirror, and assessing my past with all the good, the bad, the ugly, and the great experiences that have unfolded over many years.

Fall seven times and stand up eight.

Japanese Proverb

Chapter 5
Getting Hit Again and Again and AGAIN!

Life was good. I was operating full throttle and enjoying the new normal that I worked so hard to achieve—one that took much discipline and focus. In addition, I was consciously making different choices career-wise. Much to my surprise, I was rear-ended by distracted drivers while sitting at traffic lights in May, again in June, and yet again in August of 2014. Who does this happen to? It was like my car had a *hit me* sign on the back of it!

Getting Hit Again

The May accident was the first. I was excited to be retained by one of my favorite clients to facilitate another Articulate Leader Presentation Workshop. Twenty-eight participants from all around the country were flying into downtown Denver for this program. I left at 7:00 am to drive downtown so I could get there early and be ready to go by 8:30 am. I stopped at a traffic light and suddenly my car was rear-ended. Before I even got out of the car my neck was screaming at me in pain. I called my partner, Roni, and asked her to drive to the scene of the accident with icepacks. The driver got out of his car, apologized profusely, and said he was distracted. We called the police. Roni arrived a few minutes later and I was having trouble focusing, so Roni filled out the police report. I immediately contacted my colleague to let him know I was in an accident and would be detained so we would have a late start. I also asked James, my liaison and internal business partner for the program, to have a bottle of Advil ready for me when I arrived and a few people available to unload materials from my car as any lifting would add to the pain I was already experiencing.

There were 28 people waiting for their workshop and cancelling was not an option. As soon as the police released us, I drove downtown, practicing a breathing exercise called 6-3-6 all the way there. I went to the client's quiet room. When I felt more centered, I walked into the room and everyone clapped and smiled happily acknowledging that I had been hurt and still showed up for them. The workshop began before I even had time to focus on my reinjured neck. I put all my attention on facilitating the training for eight hours, popping Advil and putting ice packs on my neck throughout the session. I powered through the entire day. My client was so grateful that I kept this commitment. I was so touched when she sent me flowers and a thank you note on behalf of her and the class.

I reached out to Dr. Bill Borman, my chiropractor, during a break and made an appointment to see him after class ended. At 8:00 p.m. that night, Roni drove me to Bill's home office. By the time I arrived, I was in agony. Bill worked on my screaming body pain to help me through the night and next day.

We had a second day workshop to fulfill so I showed up to complete it, as it was important to me to keep my commitment. I later went through another round of cognitive testing and found out from my cognitive therapist that this car accident was a concussive event, hence another brain injury.

Getting Hit Again and Again

In the month of June, I was driving to my women's group for our bi-monthly evening get together and I forgot how to get there, even though I had driven to June Clayton's home hundreds of times in the past many years. This was a sign I really did have another brain injury. I ended up taking another route. While stopping at a light, I started to turn right, saw a car coming, and stopped just in time. In the meantime, the driver behind me was in a hurry to meet his girlfriend and did not realize I had stopped. He rear-ended me. I was barely healed up from the May accident and got hit *again!* My neck issues were exacerbated, and my body hurt. The next day, I went back to Bill, the chiropractor, and continued for many sessions afterwards.

Getting Hit Again and Again and Again

The biggest of the three hits was in August (at least I got a reprieve for one month). I was driving to facilitate a one-hour training program on behalf of a New York based company that has hired me for years as one of their Associate Trainers—a side job. I was on a major road one block from where the session was to occur, waiting again at a light, when *boom*! Everything in the car went flying, and I was quickly rocked forward and backward. Evidently an elderly attorney on the way to work was trying to get from the right lane to the left lane, but there was a car in his blind spot. He hit that car, that car hit the car in front of it, another car was hit, and *that* car hit me—it was a four-car wreck. My neck and body were injured once again. This accident was almost too much to bear. Getting hit *again*, the third time in four months, was absolutely devastating. I had another concussion (brain injury), and my cognitive functioning declined significantly.

These accidents were a tremendous setback. I became tired easily and had more difficulty with short-term memory and word retrieval than prior to May 2014. I suffered from headaches, TMJ/jaw, and neck pain, and my movements were somewhat stiff.

I ended up going back to cognitive therapy, vision therapy, neuro-physical therapy, chiropractic therapy, etc. My life as I knew it changed once again. My friends and colleagues noticed significant changes in my moods, emotions, thought processes, memory, and my ability to function as I used to function. My experience facilitating the training in Miami (Chapter 3) was one of the most painful results of this last injury. To understand these changes at a deeper level, the letters in the Addendum were written by people who knew and worked with me prior to the three accidents in 2014. They documented the changes that they witnessed in me. There was a significant impact on my health and life as I had known it, and again I was determined to do whatever it would take to reach another new normal.

As a side note: After the third accident, one of the professionals treating me recommended that I purchase a copper rod from the plumbing department at a hardware store and put it in the back of my car to prevent any other accidents. Copper is believed to be a protective trace mineral with healing properties. It is also believed to provide protection from negative energies and can be used to deflect energies. While this may sound crazy, I have been accident free since I followed this advice. The rod was completely straight when purchased; it is now bent, so I am convinced that it has been protecting me.

It became apparent that I needed to retain an attorney, as insurance company paperwork was overflowing. Phone calls from the insurance companies became a daily occurrence. Offers for a one-time pain and suffering settlement were coming my way, and the entire process was becoming overwhelming. While it would feel overwhelming to anyone who had multiple car wrecks in a four-month time frame, it was even more so for me with the body pain and the new, additional brain injuries. My friend June and I interviewed personal injury attorneys. From my perspective, we selected the very best in town, Rebecca B. Albano from the Law Office of Rebecca Albano. Rebecca and I co-wrote Chapter 6, which discusses everything I learned about litigation. I hope this will help you if you are ever in a similar situation.

Getting hit again and again and again brought me many more life lessons to learn along the way. I am grateful to be here and alive to write about them!

Let us never negotiate out of fear
but let us never fear to negotiate.
John F. Kennedy

Chapter 6
Navigating the Legal System

Litigation Through the Eyes of a Brain Injury
Survivor and Her Attorney

By Rebecca Albano, Esq.
and Joanne E. Cohen, MA, CBIS

The purpose of this Chapter is to share insights into
what was learned over a two-year time period (2014-
2016) following three assaults/hits in the spring and
summer of 2014, so that other people with brain
injuries (as well as professionals who advocate and
support them) can reflect and make the best decisions.
We will discuss how to lead a brain injury survivor
through the insurance and litigation process.

How to Select the Right Attorney for You

There are expert attorneys who exhibit and make presentations to the brain injury community, which often leads Brain Injury (BI) participants to seek them out for representation. In this chapter, we witness the litigation arena through the eyes of a brain injury survivor who actually went through this process. Selecting the right attorney is critical to your survival of the process, your sanity, and to obtaining the best results.

The first part of the selection process is to answer some important questions about legalities, such as: Does the attorney have the qualifications in the area I need? Does s/he have a proven track record? Is the attorney respected in his or her field?

We invite you to ask your potential attorney these essential questions:

- In what area of law do you specialize?

- What percentage of your practice is dedicated to personal injury, specifically, people with brain injury?

- How many people like me have you represented?

- Are you on a contingency fee or hourly fee, and what are the financial risks?

- Do I have a case to win?

- What would be your approach or philosophy to winning my case?

Do your research! Get referrals and recommendations through your network to assist you with this process.

After you have answered these questions, check in with your intuition—your gut. Intuitively, who will make you feel like you are a person in the process and not a robot.

Make your decision based upon facts *and* your intuition. The attorney-client relationship is important. It is imperative that your attorney understands brain injury, connects with you, makes you feel a part of the process, personally returns phone calls in a timely manner, and has empathy and compassion—what a novel idea!

Would your potential attorney make you feel like a partner in your case? Would you feel empowered versus disempowered? Honored versus disrespected? Listened to versus ignored? Would you feel as though you will have a say in your case and that your voice matters?

Your attorney should be centered, grounded, level-headed, smart, and caring. He or she should understand that while suffering from a brain injury, you are contending with a loss of reserves, having difficulty with fatigue and energy management (see the Emotional Reserve Model in Chapter 3, Key 10) and dealing with the emotional aspects, financial pressures, and stress.

It is extremely important to bring an advocate with you as you interview attorneys. This person should serve as your alter-ego and a voice of reason, and help you make decisions rather than making decisions for you. This person will also help you process the pros and cons of each attorney you are considering. Joanne was fortunate enough to have her friend June, a retired court reporter, assist her in the selection process.

If you select your attorney carefully, he or she will be a partner with you and stand up for you through this difficult and trying process.

The Insurance Assault

In the days after you arrive home from the accident(s), you will be inundated with paperwork and phone calls from all of the players involved, the most intense of which will be from the insurance companies—yours and the other parties'. While you are in severe pain and in an acute stage of brain injury, this process is very overwhelming and taxing on the brain, especially if you try to do it alone. (This is another reason to find an attorney to lend support.)

This stage makes it very difficult to seek appropriate treatment, heal, and get back to a new normal. Many brain injury survivors tend to want to get well quickly and may overextend themselves in an effort to do so by seeking multiple treatments and providers. Keep this in mind and seek expert assistance to select the treatments that benefit you most with the appropriate timing.

During this stage, you will be contacted with a litany of necessary documentation, including medical releases and other items that may put the insurance company on stronger footing than you. Seek out the right helpers and experts during this timeframe. You are in a vulnerable state, and insurance companies will take advantage of your vulnerability.

You most likely will be contacted by the at-fault insurance company with a pain and suffering offer, which very likely will not compensate you for your damages and may not take into account any continuing injury or treatment. Your injuries and damages may worsen or change as time goes on and as the dust settles.

Understand the limitations of your capacity at this juncture and make wise decisions in this regard. Every claim has a time limitation or statute of limitation, depending upon the type of claim and the state in which the injury occurred. Legal intricacies abound. Take a step back, breathe, and consult the appropriate professionals before making any rash decisions that you may regret later. Take the advice of your own counsel.

Process and Choices

Now let's consider the process you will go through and the decisions you will need to make. For the purposes of this book, we will go over the processes and laws of the State of Colorado; note that the law is a constantly changing body and varies by jurisdiction. Verify your rights and responsibilities with your legal counsel in your state. Again, this chapter is not intended to take the place or be representative of legal advice.

Throughout the injury process, there will be many crossroads. You will be empowered to make choices throughout this process, and you can start and stop anywhere along the way. Some of these choices include:

Do I accept the insurance company's one-time offer for pain and suffering? Do I retain an attorney? Once I retain an attorney, do we present medical damages or lost wages? What other damages have I suffered? Do I have the chance to try to settle my claim out of Court? What is a fair offer? Do I file a lawsuit or not? Do I proceed to trial, or do I stop at some point along the way?

The Litigation Process of an Injury Case

To paraphrase Shakespeare, "To litigate, or not to litigate, that is the question." If your case does not settle in the pre-litigation phase, you may be faced with the option of litigation—the process of taking legal action. The litigation process has many twists and turns along the way. Competent legal counsel can lead you through this process. The following are some relevant steps of the litigation process:

- Complaint. The initial process of filing a lawsuit involves the process of filing a complaint. The complaint alleges and details all injuries and damages that have occurred due to the negligence of the at-fault party. A legal complaint must be filed within the applicable time period of the statute of limitation.

- Answer. The civil defendant (the person or entity against whom the suit is brought) will have the opportunity to respond to the complaint in the form of a pleading called an *answer*.

- Discovery. Discovery begins shortly after the case is at issue, meaning all parties have answered and filed responsive pleadings. The discovery process varies depending upon whether your case is brought in federal or state court. Every jurisdiction is different and may have different rules and requirements. Discovery is the overarching term that describes the process of exchanging information in a civil case.

- Rule 26 disclosures. Initial Rule 26 disclosures are exchanged once the case is at issue. These disclosures involve the exchange of all information that may be helpful and/or relevant to your claim. Your friends and family members who may have information regarding your condition before and after the accident are disclosed, along with all records and all treating physicians and experts, and any other individuals with relevant information. One way to stay ahead of the discovery snowball is to start to gather this information with your attorney during the initial litigation preparation process.

- Interrogatories, requests for production of documents, and requests for admission. All of these are questions or requests that ask for relevant (and sometimes not so relevant) information to your claim. They involve a proverbial re-digging up of your life. This process can be extremely stressful. You have legal support from the staff of your legal team, but your litigation team will need you to locate the information and provide it in a timely manner to effectively litigate your claim. This process can feel invasive while you are at a vulnerable time in your life. Important documentation to provide your attorney may include police reports, injury documentation, and statements of friends, family, and physicians. You may need to retrace your steps and medical treatment to provide clarity on a particular allegation or injury. Be clear with your medical providers and keep adequate documentation on record to support your claims. Memories fade; therefore, it is vitally important to contact witnesses early and to preserve their statements.

- Depositions. A deposition is an oral examination that is recorded by way of a court reporter; it can also be recorded by a videographer. In this proceeding, you will provide testimony under oath. Although depositions take place outside of a courtroom setting, this testimony can be used against you. You must be absolutely truthful, just as you would during trial testimony. Depositions are used for fact gathering and may be taken to secure a Plaintiff's answers prior to trial. In the event a Plaintiff's answers change at trial, a Plaintiff can be impeached for untruthful testimony. (More on how to prepare for a deposition on page 172.)

How to Prepare for a Deposition

You have a brain injury (or injuries) and ask yourself, *How can I do this? How can I remember what I need to remember and survive the process?* The *only* way out is through.

There are two levels of preparation for your deposition. Your attorney should properly prepare you to be deposed. The first level of preparation involves the factual and procedural preparation. The second and equally important aspect is the emotional preparation. It is very important that you listen to the advice of your counsel during this phase.

It is also very important that you, the deponent (the person being deposed) is adequately prepared for the procedural aspects of the deposition, as well as the subject matter it may cover. An attorney may spend several hours preparing you for the process. Ask questions if you do not understand or recall information that may be sought. If you do not remember the answer to the question posed, testify truthfully that you do not recall or know the information sought rather than testifying inaccurately. Do not feel badly or beat yourself up for what you cannot remember.

Keep in mind that any information you bring into the proceeding may become discoverable (that is, able to be requested by the opposing party through a legal process, such as a subpoena). Therefore, it is important that your testimony reflects your best recollection.

It is vital that you testify truthfully and authentically through your deposition process. Resist the temptation to give long responses to questions asked. Keep in mind that less is more. Just answer the questions without adding extra information. It is absolutely okay to answer with a simple *yes, no,* or *I do not remember.* Joanne received this advice from her court reporter friend June, prior to going into the deposition and this was extremely helpful while being deposed.

Depositions tend to trigger emotions and bring back unpleasant memories. At times, they can make you, the victim, feel judged, attacked, and disempowered. Remember that you are dealing with attorneys who are *not* your friends; many will chip away at your cognitive fatigue. They *are* just doing their job. They may make you feel like you're in the wrong, their questions may exhaust you, and you may feel intimidated, persecuted, and assaulted. You have to have the stomach to go through this process, and then decide whether you wish to move forward with the remainder of the litigation process. At the end of each day, make every effort to leave what you went through in the room, knowing that you did your very best.

It is important to protect yourself energetically. Whatever your faith or spirituality or religion, tap into your spiritual place of strength. If the opposing lawyer comes after you about an intricacy or item that you cannot remember, and you do not seem to be on equal footing, find your emotional strength to overcome what feels like the unfairness of the process. Focus on your ability; embrace the dis of disability.

It can be frustrating if an opposing attorney references an item that you are not privy to or that you do not recall. Stay calm. Answer carefully, truthfully, and remember that it's okay to say, I do not know.

Joanne recalls a scenario during her deposition where the opposing attorney asked a question about an intricacy in her medical records. She mustered the courage to state, "Well, I am a brain injury survivor and am doing my best to recollect without notes… YOU have the records in front of you. If that's what the doctor said, then I would go with that!" And she remembers smiling, thinking of the irony, that a brain injury survivor like herself could be grilled regarding these intricacies without records or notes to reference while the opposing legal counsel had all of their notes in front of them. Per legal advice, Joanne would risk the discoverability of her notes by bringing them into the proceeding. It presents a challenging scenario for a brain injury survivor to recall events and details without any notes.

If you are already in a place of trauma, the opposing party may re-victimize you. Be ready. If you believe in yourself, trust the truth, be authentic, and protect yourself energetically—you *will* thrive. Following completion of the deposition, while it is easier said than done, do *not* beat yourself up. You must know that you did the best you could do. Continue to trust your helpers as the process progresses.

Mediation

Some judges will require the occurrence of a mediation process and some will not. The parties may agree that mediation may be helpful to foster resolution of the case. Mediation involves third-party intervention to try to resolve the dispute or case. Mediation is different from arbitration and may occur in a more informal or private corporate setting outside of a courthouse.

A mediator may discuss the strengths and weaknesses of your case. This can be valuable trial preparation and may reveal important arguments of the opposing party. A mediator may ask for an update regarding the condition of your physical or emotional injury. It is important that you feel comfortable with the selected mediator and that you are not pressured into making any decisions that you do not feel comfortable or equipped to make.

Numbers or terms of settlement may be discussed, and a mediator may take several trips back and forth between the parties throughout the day. If a settlement is reached in mediation, this may be the end of the case. The parties must agree to the necessary terms to end the case at this juncture.

Be aware that the mediation process can feel one-sided. The opposing party may try to make you feel wrong or unethical. He or she may provide a low-ball offer, and you may decide to stick it out, accept the offer, or to leave and move forward and go to trial. That decision, that crossroad, is yours to make.

> *Litigation is the pursuit of practical ends,*
> *not a game of chess.*
> *Felix Frankfurter, Supreme Court Judge*

Trial

If your case does not settle during mediation, you will need to decide whether you will proceed to trial. Trial is the ultimate crossroad during the litigation process. It is a similar process to the deposition but involves testimony on the stand and the presentation of all evidence. Trial, depending upon jurisdiction and other intricacies, may involve a jury, or it may be a bench or judge trial. The result will represent some level of finality, though appealable.

Trials can be extremely expensive and risky ventures, depending upon the facts and/or witnesses necessary to adequately present the case. Trials involve serious risk, including the potential award of costs and/or fees against you if you do not succeed. Your counsel may spend thousands of dollars attempting to secure your verdict, and you may very well owe these expenses at the end.

Trial can be a risky and emotional process. A claimant may feel scrutinized or put on trial, even as the injured party. The claimant may be judged or painted as a bad or immoral person. His or her indiscretions or prior health conditions will be widely publicized and highlighted in bright neon lights for the jury.

However, the bright spot at the end of the tunnel *may* very well be that the jury *gets it!* The jury *may* see the injustice, the insanity, and they, the deciders, the helpers can make it right. Do you have the stomach to go to court? Do you have the support from your attorney, family, and friends? Do you have adequate emotional and psychological support during the preparation and trial process?

Keep in mind that the more complicated your legal claim is, the more items may need to be proved at trial. For instance, in a fact pattern involving multiple accidents or losses, or a significant preexisting injury status, the opposing party will provide a vast and unending level of blame or finger-pointing. He or she may try to create confusion or uncertainty. Expert witnesses may be hired that will be paid large sums of money to testify against your best interests.

Your trial won't be anything close to what you've seen on television. The risks and potential results are real, so make sure you understand them!

Lessons Learned Through the School of Hard Knocks

What will a trip through the civil justice system teach you as an injured person? You may feel at the end of the process that you've learned about the abuse of the system. You may feel that the system is biased or one-sided. You may learn that the only way to force justice is with a jury. You may learn that there's not always a fully accessible or fair justice system. You may learn more about yourself than you ever knew. You may learn the extent of your resiliency; you may learn a lesson in optimism or acceptance. And you will most likely learn that no amount of money can bring your health back if it was lost.

Most important, you will learn that life is still happening during litigation. It does not stop; it doesn't even take a brief pause. Instead, life proceeds full steam ahead with a new and ever-presenting sideshow for you to deal with. Your children will grow, your parents will age, and your health may fade further.

The world keeps turning while the wheels of justice turn incredibly slower. You'll learn patience, perseverance, and strength. You'll learn that it's okay to accept your case ending at any point. Getting hit, getting up, moving beyond...you *can* move from surviving to thriving with the goal of becoming whole once again after the litigation process.

An Outpouring of Emotions

By the end of a long mediation, Joanne decided to accept the opposing party's best offer, which was lower than she expected/wanted rather than to move forward and proceed to trial. Her vulnerable and raw stream of consciousness the morning after the mediation sums up her true feelings:

Tears…Raw feelings and emotions are pouring out of my soul. Feelings…happy, sad, exhausted, relieved, glad…anger, gratitude, grace, feelings of disgrace…did I sell out? Or, to thine own self be true? Following my intuition and gut and while I am feeling blue…I feel relieved…I feel raw …feelings and emotions oozing out of my soul…I feel peace. So many feelings and emotions at once woke me from sleep in the darkness of night. How does one make sense of something that is what it is?

Is the *justice* system just? Or is it the just-*ice* system. As the group Foreigner sings, "It is cold as ICE, we must sacrif-*ice*, I know…. I know…." yes I *really* know…."

I am resilient. Was this *really* about money? Justice? What is right? Fair? Did I want my day in court? (not!) Or was I paying attention to the energy? Money comes from unexpected sources, and according to my spiritual beliefs, how things look are not always how they *look*… out of the depths of despair, out of challenges, comes the rising of the Phoenix, comes good, comes light, it is all good….

I have learned that there are no accidents. Each one, while painful, inconvenient, draining, adding to additional chronic pain, additional concussive events/ brain injury…each one deepening my perspective… each one leading me to ask, *what can I learn from this and how can I help others with or without brain injury to maneuver through a justice system that does not feel just?* Attorneys representing guilty, distracted drivers… those attorneys who suck off the misfortune of others and make a case against the victim, no matter what the cost, to save their precious insurance company from doing the right thing…motivated by greed, manipulation of the system, and doing whatever it takes to take the victim down, to be in-humane, and to do whatever it takes to *win*…how do these people look at themselves in the mirror? My attorney, on the other hand, was kind, always listened, was 100 percent engaged with me, my case, my providers...my attorney is in the business of helping her clients, my attorney has heart, soul, is caring, wants to do the right thing, and is in the business to help others and then be paid vs. those attorneys who are in the business just for the money....

They say I present myself well...that I am *too* highly functioning...they say minor/low impact accidents did not cause this individual (me), for all appearances, to be damaged. They say the jury won't buy it...they say the jury won't believe there was enough of an impact to cause brain injury, discounting professionals— cognitive therapist and testing, neuro-psych testing and therapist, physiatrist, physical therapist, dentist, chiropractor...letters from colleagues and friends (witnesses) who knew me prior to and after the three rear-end collisions caused by three men and according to Colorado law, rear-ended me and are negligent. *They* are negligent and yet their attorney's case is that I don't know how to drive at a yield sign... *really*? They believe they have a strong case to win in court—they do not think a jury will care or understand the impact of these three accidents and its effects. While the evidence is in my favor, would the jury believe it or not? The pictures of property damage to our two automobiles does not reflect the damage to me, however, will the jury of my six peers understand and buy this truth? At the end of the day, we had two options:

Option 1: Go deeper into the trenches and get their experts involved—an MD and psychiatrist paid off by the insurance companies to say there is nothing wrong with me, that it's all in my head (approximately $14,000); a biomechanical engineer (approximately $7,000); perhaps one of their neuropsychologists to look at the extensive reports my neuropsychologist wrote and spin the results in favor of the insurance company (approximately $5,000)—*and*, if I lose the case, I would have the honor of paying all those expenses and more of up to at least $50,000.

Option 2: See their low-balled bottom line and settle. Part of me wanted to go to court out of principle… part of me wanted this to just be over so I could move on with my life and put all of it behind me…did I really want to add another 4-6 plus months of stress, uncertainty, lack of control of who is on the jury and our burden of proof that the accidents caused additional brain injuries? I called a lifeline, my sister-in-law, Debbie Cohen, and my attorney and I spent 40 minutes on the phone with her for her opinion/viewpoint…I thought about my life force, my energy, and is money really worth the risk of debt if we lost? Is money really worth my life being on hold for another year or more? Is money worth participating in a trial where I will hear negativity, lies, things that are *just* not the truth about me? After deep contemplation and listening to my intuition and gut, I decided to settle for a very small amount and be grateful.

When all was said and done, and when the amount of money offered was so low…I revisited a previous discussion and a new line of business is born. In addition to doing my presentation, *Litigation through the eyes of a brain injury survivor,* we discussed an additional contribution I can make from all I have learned/experienced while going through this challenging litigation process that led to settling vs. going to court. I birthed a seed planted by my optometrist—

my becoming a consultant (coach) to deal with clients who may be difficult, who are stressed, who could use coaching on how to be more likeable and how to present themselves during a deposition, mediation, and trial—a trial consultant…an expert witness consultant…a plaintiffs' consultant…See? How things looked going into mediation yesterday (the dollar amount we wanted) and what came out of the day (a business where I use my wealth of knowledge to assist injured people going through the same process) was the real gift of going through everything the last two years and four months. Who would have thunk it?

Now I can move on…the energy has opened…my tears are of relief, of compassion for myself and for others, of excitement for a brighter future of living my passion and supporting others in this new way. Perhaps this is why it all happened? I don't know what I don't know…what I do know is that today is a new day, litigation is behind me, I have learned so much and law of attraction principles tell me to focus on what I want, not what I don't want, and I *want* to take this experience, put the bad stuff behind me and focus on what's to come now and in the future.

I received a text from my attorney after spending the day together in mediation: "You were an inspiration today...Thank you for being a light in the dark." Tears...more tears...all leading to joy, goodness, inner strength, love, forgiveness, leaving the past in the past, living in the now moment, and looking forward to the future....there are no accidents—they are opportunities to grow, to heal, to pay to others the generosity and kindness experienced along the way to others...and to add whatever *heat* I can to those in their process of the just*ice* system. And so, it is...

As you can see, Joanne decided during the mediation process to focus on what she learned from this process so that she could help others as a trial coach/consultant.

Attorney Testimonial

Joanne received the following testimonial written by an attorney whose client was awarded $500,000 by a jury. This flowed from her work as a coach on a traumatic brain injury trial. The work was inspired by her own experiences as a traumatic brain injury survivor and personal injury plaintiff.

> Ms. Cohen acted as a trial coach and consultant on a complicated mild traumatic brain injury case in Colorado, providing invaluable skill and support for our client and our firm. Ms. Cohen's insight into mild traumatic brain injury provided tremendous assistance in preparing the client for testimony and assisting her through the stress of trial.

> Ms. Cohen evidenced strong communication skills and was able to foster a relationship with the client that was second to none. Ms. Cohen fostered trust with our team and our client and provided tangible stress relief throughout the process for our client. Prior to trial, Ms. Cohen provided hours of instruction to our client regarding the client's testimony, demeanor, dress and stress and anxiety management techniques.

Ms. Cohen is particularly gifted at working with clients with traumatic brain injury and/or post-traumatic stress disorder, however, her years of training permit her the ability to be an invaluable source in any case whether proceeding to deposition, mediation, arbitration or trial. Ms. Cohen has an incredible talent and drive to customize her work to best fit the needs of the client and the firm by way of her attentiveness to detail and hard work to understand the case and the needs of the parties involved. Ms. Cohen's attendance at the extensive and lengthy jury trial was instrumental in assisting us to achieve a successful and unexpectedly high verdict with interest.

Ms. Cohen assisted our client with body language, dress for trial and with establishing an emotional presence and likability that would help the jury to understand the client's plight and injury in an effective and positive way. During trial preparation meetings, Ms. Cohen was influential in focusing our client on the areas that needed additional assistance to flourish at trial. Ms. Cohen also provided our client with support and important information to assist with fatigue and energy management during trial and the weeks leading up to it.

It is not surprising that Ms. Cohen is such a talented trial coach and consultant given her experience coaching and speaking over the years, specifically with a focus on providing information for people with brain injuries through CTAT, LLC (Coaching, Training, and Transformation), and the Brain Injury Hope Foundation (BIHF). Ms. Cohen has been coaching and assisting the brain injury population for more than a decade and her recent services could not have been more helpful nor more valuable.

Summary

We hope this chapter is informative for anyone considering and/or needing assistance navigating the legal process. The key is to find proper representation—somebody who will be your advocate, someone who will partner with you, and an attorney who understands brain injury and is familiar with the professionals who serve the brain injury community.

In life there is loss and grief and we can continually recreate ourselves and embrace our new normal.
Rita Coalson and Joanne Cohen

Chapter 7
Overcoming Grief and Loss after Getting Hit...Again!

Grief Through the Eyes of a Brain Injury
Survivor and Her Grief Therapist

By Rita D. Coalson, MA, LPC, NCC
and Joanne E. Cohen, MA, CBIS

Getting Hit AGAIN

On September 27, 2016, litigation ended following three car accidents resulting in two additional concussive events (traumatic brain injuries) for Joanne. On September 28, 2016, in the middle of the night, Joanne wrote the stream of consciousness essay in Chapter 6 as she processed the damage caused by the automobile accidents and her disappointment with the legal system. Sadly, she was unaware that she was about to get hit yet *again* in an even more traumatic way.

Five days later, Roni, Joanne's partner of 21 years, went to the doctor for a periodic wellness physical. One of the blood tests carried ominous information. Joanne and Roni were shocked to find out that Roni would be diagnosed with acute myeloblastic leukemia (AML) and given one to three months to live. Joanne barely had time to catch her breath from the trauma of litigation when she found herself struggling to comprehend what would become the biggest and most profound challenge of her life—losing her partner and best friend to a quick-moving terminal disease that devastated their hopes for the future.

After receiving the diagnosis, they both moved from shock to acceptance, with Joanne quickly shifting gears to become her helper, caregiver, support person, friend, driver, and advocate. When the end finally materialized, Joanne held Roni in her arms as she slipped away and took her last breath with their dear friend Cindy lending support. Joanne would later memorialize the moment as the biggest honor and privilege one could have. It was also the most profound heartbreak of her life.

Swallowed in grief, Joanne gradually began to realize that the results of this major life loss and the grief process that ensued would affect her as had her prior acute brain injuries. Many of the emotional and sensory effects of TBI were mirrored in the pronounced disturbances experienced in grieving the loss of her loved one. Symptoms included fatigue, sleep disturbance, memory loss, changes in comprehension, speed of processing, changes in emotions and moods, decreased attention and focus, and increased irritability.

Joanne entered and was part of a club that she had not chosen to belong to: the Mourners Club. This was not the first time Joanne dealt with the death of significant people in her life. When she was 25 years old, she lost a dear friend, Jimmy Dinolfo, to leukemia—the first time someone in her age group had passed away. The loss of her father, Harvey, in 1989 and her mother, Doris in 2011 were also devastating. When we lose both parents, many of us may feel like orphans and question our own mortality.

The assault on one's sense of safety from just one trauma can be debilitating. The cumulative effect of multiple emotional and physical traumas over a period of time is devastating. However, this was Joanne's new life. She had little choice but to consciously work toward another new normal and another new Joanne.

What Is Grief

To Joanne, it became obvious that there were parallels in both path and experience between grieving the loss associated with having multiple brain injuries and grieving the loss of a loved one, Joanne's partner. Here, we'll compare those similarities and focus on the grieving process in general.

Clinically, grief can be defined as a normal, appropriate, and involuntary reaction/response to a loss. Grieving is the experience of loss and causes an end or change to what we've known up to the point of loss. It can manifest itself physically, psychologically, intellectually, socially, and spiritually. Grief and its outward expression, mourning, is a process, not a discrete event. Let us reiterate: grief is a process.

As a grief therapist, Rita has counseled clients from many walks of life and has confirmed that grief is universal, messy, and *not* for wimps. Rita tells a story of a male client who sat before her revealing that his family was concerned about his way of grieving. Specifically, his family had told him that, in their opinion, he was not grieving properly. As Rita and her client talked, this father of a deceased child explained that he felt obliged to remain stoic in the face of this heart wrenching loss for the sake of his family. In his mind, it was necessary that he remain a rock that others could lean on for support. After weeks of counseling, the father came to the realization that it was okay for him to grieve outwardly as well as inwardly. And that he could do that without relinquishing his role as family protector.

Working through the pain of grief means that the bone-crushing sadness will need to be expressed outwardly. Do you need to give yourself permission to grieve? At times, you may even feel as though you are going crazy and that these feelings may soon become unbearable. This is natural and healthy. What is not healthy is to stuff these feelings down, acting as if they are not real. Over time, through expression of these feelings, you will regain a semblance of control and equilibrium. Similarly, brain injuries may also produce these horrible feelings. The same fear, anxiety, and anger may be present for those with brain injuries as occurs with those grieving a death. TBI grief is just as messy and debilitating as relationship loss. Just know that it is okay to grieve *any* loss you're experiencing and that failure to work through the pain can lead to unresolved grief, which will manifest itself in unexpected and undesirable ways.

Rita and Joanne feel that, when it comes to grief and its outward expression, the sanitized culture that we live in makes it difficult for mourners to feel accepted. Rita uses the term *sanitized* to emphasize the superficial aspects presented by a culture where social media in all of its visible manifestations demands we constantly measure ourselves; that we forever judge our adequacy. Grief is messy. The expression of grief is often ugly. There is little allowance for grieving and the accompanying negativity and raw emotion in a grief and conflict avoidant society. Grieving the loss of persons, jobs, health, personality, or diminished cognitive abilities is made more difficult because of society's failure to understand and support those in the throes of grieving. As the poet Carl Sandburg once said, "Life is like an onion. You peel it off one layer at a time, and sometimes you weep."[4] As you go through the onion layers of grief, you adjust to each layer and weep.

This apparent lack of empathy for grieving people is further understood as we consider that in our society people maintain different perceptions of what grief is and isn't. There is scant evidence of culturally acceptable methods of grieving. For the most part, we are left alone to work it out for ourselves. Two adult siblings came to Rita reflecting that they were struggling with how each of them was grieving the death of their mother. The brother explained that his sister never talked about their mother, rarely showed any emotion regarding their loss, and had gone back to work immediately after their mother died. She was a successful career woman, and her work was her passion. The sister was frustrated that her brother talked continuously about their mother often resulting in awkward emotional outbursts.

Rita and her clients had to discuss the fact that each person has a unique view of how one should grieve. Conversely, humans also look outside of themselves for confirmation that their personal behavior is correct, wanting not only acceptance but confirmation from others. Both siblings were grieving, each in their own way. After some discussion, each began to understand that mourning is personal, and each person's grieving behaviors are valid and need to be respected.

Grief is an experience like no other human event. The terror and emptiness comes in many forms and intensities, like a monster on the doorstep of your mind delivering chaos, anxiety, sadness, and emptiness at unpredictable intervals. To handle it properly, we must be in the moment as much as possible. Further, everyone appears to grieve differently based upon the moment in which they find themselves. As Hospice Affiliate Nina Hart pointed out to Joanne, "Grief is like a boiling pot, and no one knows what pops up."

Characteristics of Grief

The death of a loved one rocks your world to the core. Loss often requires you to examine who you are and your ability to feel secure in a world that has changed so suddenly. The same is true for people with brain injuries. You often feel out of control, vulnerable, and full of raw emotions. The world as you know it isn't the same, and you may no longer feel as safe as you once thought.

There are many ways grief manifests itself through mourning. Some of the facets of grief affect the physical, emotional, cognitive, and behavioral aspects of one's life. Physically, grievers may experience fatigue, gastrointestinal issues, sleep problems, restlessness, and more. Emotionally, feelings of frustration, emptiness, anger, loneliness, and despair are common. Cognitively, you can experience memory loss, confusion, and a lack of control. Behaviorally, grieving involves dealing with crying, social withdrawal, or uncontrolled periods of nervousness and excessive activity.

The differing effects of grief often come in oscillating waves. We often become discouraged when we thought we have made progress only to find one day that we are re-experiencing the acuteness of yesterday's grief. Don't lose heart. This is natural. Take the waves as they come, and reach out for help and support where available, expanding your support system as your grieving process dictates. Experiencing grief is a lot like walking into an ocean; as you move forward, wave after wave slams into you, often knocking you down as well as backward. Gradually, however, you will make your way beyond the breakers and life will return to a semblance of equilibrium. Those experiencing brain injuries will also have to deal with periodic setbacks in their grieving of the person they were before the trauma.

Grief Categories

One of the primary tasks facing researchers is the goal to categorize behaviors within a defined, measurable set of characteristics. In an attempt to identify and explain the grieving process, inherent characteristics have been grouped into a category called Type. Two of the many types of grief, Disenfranchised Grief and Secondary Loss, have been established and are common to both those grieving the loss of a person and those suffering from a TBI. Here's a closer look at each type.

Disenfranchised Grief is characterized as grief that is shaded by social discomfort or unacceptability. For example, a man who grieves the death of an ex-wife, a woman who laments the loss of her husband in the face of a life sentence, or a person who grieves their loss of effectiveness at work following a head trauma are all scenarios where society may refrain from authorizing the grieving process due to the shame or ambiguity associated with each situation. The divorce is in the past, prisoners don't deserve grief, and brain injuries are often invisible to those looking on. Disenfranchised grief happens more than we wish. Not many people are modeled healthy grieving; therefore, grief associated with a loss is neither fully understood nor accepted. From an outsiders view, mourners can appear as frustratingly inefficient, absent, and antisocial.

We believe society as a whole values people who are productive, efficient, and can perform well. Society's failure to accurately understand the characteristics of and hurdles faced by mourners creates a disturbing headwind frustrating the natural processing of grief. We encourage people with brain injuries to create an effective support system, such as the Survivor Series. The Brain Injury Hope Foundation (BIHF) resurrected and implemented the series in 2018. The goal of the series is to help those bravely adjusting with a BI to have a place to not just strive, but to thrive and be part of a community that understands them—a sense of community and a sense of belonging to eventually achieve the life they desire.

We believe and, in fact, highly recommend that those in the brain injury community seek out support groups to help create a new normal so they do not feel so alone and isolated. It is imperative to network to find an effective support system in your community.

That's what has been created through the monthly Colorado BIHF's Survivor Series which provides resources for brain injury survivors, professional providers, family members, caregivers, partners/ significant others, and friends whose important services are funded by grants. (To read blogs associated with

these events, go to braininjuryhopefoundation.org/
blog-2/.) The Survivor Series continues to be valuable
to our brain injury community and supports all of us
as we move from striving and surviving to *thriving*.

Secondary Loss is another type of grief and is
experienced when one becomes aware that an outcome
has changed as a result of a primary loss; brain damage
or loss of a significant other is classed as a primary
loss. For example, following the death of a significant
other the bereaved is faced with paying bills previously
handled by the deceased. The survivor is not a detail-
oriented person and the accounting tasks naturally
landed in her partner's lap. Another example might be
the recognition that one can no longer get through
a social setting without their outgoing partner. The
primary loss is the core functionality (due to a TBI)
or the significant other who is no longer present. The
secondary loss is the event, behavior, or experience
that collaterally is lost as a result of the primary loss.
Another secondary loss may be the insufficiency of
your existing support system. Prior to the loss, your
friends and family provided the help that you needed
to negotiate life as it was. The current loss, however, is

such that your support system is ill-equipped to help as they often cannot adequately relate to your new situation. The loss of one's support system is significant and only becomes fully understood as time passes. The reconstruction of an effective support system will have a positive impact on the overall grieving process. "The friend who can be silent with us in a moment of despair or confusion, who can stay with us in an hour of grief and bereavement, who can tolerate not knowing…not healing, not curing…that is a friend who cares."[5] Secondary loss affects people with brain injuries just as it affects those who have experienced the death of a loved one. A brain injury is the primary loss; the everyday challenges you face while trying to adjust to your new way of life are the secondary losses.

Support systems can fail a griever in many ways. One particularly painful situation occurs when friends and or family members attempt to influence the griever to return to the person they were prior to the loss. The griever is immeasurably frustrated at this attempt as no one wants the original you more than the griever themselves.

Considering secondary losses associated with brain injuries, the effects can be more acute, such as those involving physical functionality. Behaviors that were once taken for granted can now become physically dangerous. For example, Joanne once didn't realize she was driving 40 mph in a 25-mph school zone and received a $200 speeding ticket. Unfortunately, she didn't realize at the time that she was in a brain fog due to the loss of her loved one, her brain injury, and the grief associated with both. When you're in an acute stage of brain injury, be especially mindful when driving. You *think* you're clear and focused but in reality, you may not be.

Joanne also experienced a parallel parking incident during this time. Prior to the latest injury, she'd considered herself to be a skilled parallel parker since the age of 16. While parallel parking after the loss of Roni she hit a truck parked in front of her, which caused $2,000 of damage to her car. Fortunately, there was no damage to the truck.

These types of situations are wake up calls to be taken seriously so we don't hurt ourselves or others. Joanne embraced these calls and made every effort to drive only while feeling focused and alert. Brain fog from injury or grief can affect many areas of your life, including mistaking salt for sugar in a recipe and ending up with a culinary disaster!

A Grief Model

According to J. William Worden, Ph.D., there are four tasks of mourning[6] that are parallel to experiencing grief and experiencing a brain injury. The four tasks that can facilitate the grieving process are acceptance of the reality of the loss, embracing the pain accompanying the loss, embracing your world as it exists without that which was lost, and finally to, in Worden's words "relocate" the loss from the present, allowing it to recede into the past. The thinking behind Worden's Tasks of Mourning, and the suggestions of others who labor to understand the grieving process, lies in the belief that unprocessed grief is itself a destructive force. Failure to adequately process grief can have detrimental effects over the rest of one's life.

Working on these four tasks is understood to be addressed in a fluid, rather than a step-wise manner. The characteristic of "fluidity" indicates that the associated tasks and goals can and must be addressed in a random or cyclical fashion, not unlike a bee dipping randomly into the flowers in a field. There is no particular order in which flowers are visited by the bee. Likewise, there is no restraint on the bee visiting the same flower more than once. Eventually, though, the bee will gather nectar from all the flowers. With respect to the tasks of mourning, you will often revisit a task as you experience moments that trigger emotions you previously addressed. Dipping back and forth into this or that emotional area as one moves through the tasks associated with the grieving process is not uncommon.

The first task of grieving is to accept the reality of the loss. This conscious acceptance will give you a strong foundation upon which a new life can be built. We stated earlier that grief is not for wimps. This step of acceptance is immensely difficult and will take some time. It will also be intense at times and will require escape until a revisit is possible. One way to accomplish this task is by telling your story to others. There is a benefit to hearing your own words confirm the loss. Additionally, hearing others speak of the loss will also work in favor of your eventual acceptance of the new reality.

Stories recounting past events and interactions with the loved one who has died will serve to present the new reality while also preserving the memories shared with the deceased. These stories will help you reaffirm your sense of identity and relationship to your loved one while simultaneously bringing the deceased closer to you and reducing your sense of loss and isolation.

This task applies equally to those who have had a brain injury. Recounting memories of how you functioned prior to the BI and articulating your current functionality will help you move in the direction of acceptance of a new reality. For one BI survivor, it took two years for her to realize that she was mourning the loss of who she had been prior to the injury coupled with anxiety as to who she would become. Once she embraced her story and accepted the reality of her situation, she turned a corner regarding her depression and grief, allowing her zest for life to reignite. It is important to realize there is a mourning process, and you cannot sweep it under the rug, nor can you hide from its fury—it needs to be acknowledged and dealt with to move forward.

The second task of mourning is embracing the pain accompanying the loss. This means giving yourself permission to cry, get angry, be completely frustrated, and feel the guilt that accompanies grief. Let yourself experience and accept every emotion that comes along. Doris Sanders, a BI survivor, colleague, and friend of Joanne's, feels that she lost her life as she knew it when her brain injury occurred. She finished climbing mountains on all seven continents prior to the occurrence of debilitating brain injuries. Doris was training to be the oldest woman to climb Mt. Everest for her 70th birthday. She was a runner, very athletic, a 25-mile-per-day backpacker, very social, outgoing, etc. As a result of her brain injuries, she can no longer associate in large crowds due to the lights, the noise, and the colors that become disorienting. She does not go to parties due to her hearing that the brain injury affected. She also can do very little exercise. Doris tried to cope with her brain injury by using maxims, such as, *when there is a will, there is a way,* and *mind over matter.* She felt that was counterproductive and did not support her dealing with her anger, guilt, and frustration due to her altered life, nor did she grieve or mourn the deep losses from her previous life prior to the brain injury. After five years of therapy, Doris finally learned that for her, anger and grief are the same things. Doris eventually acquired the ability to deal with the grief of the losses she was mourning and feel the feelings associated with her losses and her life as it used to be.

Each mourner will experience their own level of physical, behavioral, and emotional pain associated with their specific loss. However, in terms of working through the mourning process, it is of great importance that one does not behave in such a way as to avoid or inhibit the experiencing of the pain of grief. Sadly, our society has a tendency to be grief avoidant in that outward expression of grief often makes those around the mourner uncomfortable. So much so that one's family and friends often encourage the mourner to end their grieving after a short period of time; a period of time that prohibits working on this task. A mourner, upon hearing comments that they should be over their grief is often motivated to short-circuit this task by denying or ignoring their pain.

It is vitally important to continue to work on this task. To that end, it is important to find a support system where there is the proper understanding of the grieving process and where one is allowed to experience and express their pain as long as necessary. An experienced Grief Counselor can be invaluable to the mourner struggling with feelings of inappropriateness or weakness in the face of their continuing experience of the pain of loss.

The third task is to adjust to an environment in which the deceased is absent. In the case of brain-injured persons, this is an environment in which your cognitive or physical capacity has been altered. Negotiating a changed world is a fearful and frustrating task. While this task differs depending upon the type of loss one is experiencing, it is safe to say that this is the most physical of the four tasks. For example, in most relationships, the daily living tasks tend to arrange themselves according to the abilities of each person in the relationship. The one who is meticulous usually is responsible for the record keeping efforts: paying bills, arranging social events, etc. Technical or mechanical duties may also fall to one of the two who is so inclined. With the loss of a person, you are now left with the duties previously performed by your partner. Similarly, TBI's often require that you re-learn physical or mental abilities that are no longer available to you. In some cases, outside help needs to be solicited to get a job done. Similarly, there are external, internal, and spiritual adjustments that must be confronted. External adjustments include how you're affected every day. Internal adjustments refer to your sense of self. Spiritual adjustments relate to how your situation affects your beliefs, values, and assumptions about the world.

Liz Sommers, a BI survivor since 2017 and a colleague and friend of Joanne's and blogger for the BIHF Survivor Series, shared a story about the holidays. One day, she reached the point where she embraced the reality of who she is now. Confidently, she accepted herself; this is the new me! She then posed the question, *How can*

I make my life work? Liz was inspired by the nativity story where Joseph and Mary had to trust and believe that they would be provided for as they went to Egypt. Once Liz was brain-injured with an invisible disability and achieved some financial income, she knew she would be taken care of as she continued her recovery. Her spiritual teacher taught her that you know, you trust, and you believe the spiritual component. Liz always identified herself as a sports journalist and now embraces herself as a survivor who is reinventing her life; hence, her sense of self. She continues to explore what she calls the *new me* and is moving forward with confidence. Externally, Liz is embracing her deficits while exploring new avenues as a spiritual writer and teacher that fit who she is today, her new normal.

The fourth task is to relocate the loss from the present, allowing it to recede into the past. This step involves emotionally engaging your new situation, embracing a new way of thinking, embracing the new way you invest in your life and the lives of others, and adjusting to your new normal. This task encourages the mourner to gradually shift you focus, in terms of daily activities, away from the deceased and on to people and events that remain in one's sphere. Joanne learned to adjust to living alone, to feeling safe again, and learning new coping skills. She also learned to adjust to her new responsibilities, the responsibilities of her beloved, and the mutual responsibilities previously shared with her partner.

Prior to Roni's death, Joanne and her partner divided and conquered when it came to running errands, doing the laundry, grocery shopping, preparing dinner and cleaning up afterwards, etc. At first, taking on all of these responsibilities diminished Joanne's reserves, leading to cognitive fatigue, sadness, and a lack of energy. In time, however, Joanne eventually learned to embrace and adjust to her new life and her new normal.

Styles of Grief

Doka and Martin explain that there are two styles of grievers: Instrumental and Intuitive. The *instrumental griever* tends to focus on practical matters and problem-solving, tending to get involved with tasks and projects utilizing cognitive and physical activities. They approach loss as a problem to be solved. Alternatively, the *intuitive griever* tends to focus on experiencing and expressing emotion. They focus on their feelings and involve themselves with the expression of their emotions associated with the loss. Instrumental grievers have been responsible for creating some very important organizations over the years. One notable non-profit organization, Mothers Against Drunk Driving (MADD), began through the efforts of a mother whose daughter was killed by a drunk driver. The Richard Lambert Foundation is another non-profit organization that serves its community, and which was founded by a mother who lost her young son. Both of these organizations and many others have risen from the ashes of grief to become vital centers of support for those most in need. These and other projects that have their beginnings in the pain and suffering associated with loss are a living testimony to the strength found in the human condition.

Another example of instrumental grieving was exhibited when Joanne directed a couple of improvement projects at her home including having her entire home painted on the inside and a kitchen remodel. Additionally, she reorganized her garage and basement with the help of her friend, John. The reorganization involved letting go of Roni's clothes, collectables, and books, along with 21 years of their personal belongings and some of her mother's clothes and items. These efforts triggered a flood of emotions resulting in acute grief in addition to cognitive, physical, and emotional fatigue. Keep in mind, however, that the assumption of tasks or projects in no way implies that the instrumental style of grieving is any less painful or emotionally debilitating. On the contrary, these accomplishments of instrumental grievers point to the fact that sadness and pain can be strong motivators.

Intuitive grievers are what most people consider the classic griever; one who exhibits visual expressions of despair, periods of crying and shaking, depression, anger, etc. In some cultures, intuitive grieving involves public wailing, rending one's clothes, and fainting.

It is very important to realize that grievers seldom behave solely as either intuitive or instrumental grievers. More commonly, grievers are a combination of these two styles, sliding back and forth along a continuum between the two extremes. As an example, a female client sat across from Rita distraught because she was not able to control her emotions. It had been a year and a half since her husband had died, and she had assumed that she was well on her way through the grieving process. Since the untimely death of her husband, she had been busy handling the many details of her husband's estate, including the business that he owned. Her friends were amazed at how well she appeared to be doing. Suddenly, she was inexplicably overcome with emotional and physical grief. She felt like she was falling apart. She wasn't sleeping well and was plagued by an ever-present feeling of loneliness. Rita spent some time discussing her initial instrumental behavior following her husband's death in order that she realize that her projects and tasks were, more or less, thrust upon her based on her circumstances. Nonetheless, her embrace of the tasks served to limit her exposure to the emotional consequences of her loss until the present. Now, she will begin to process her loss from an intuitive perspective. Armed with her understanding of why she was experiencing her grief in a normal, albeit postponed, time frame, she braced herself for the next phase of her grief journey.

At many points during a griever's journey, there are momentary glimpses of having come through to the other side. That perhaps they are over the acute pain. However, just as suddenly, they find themselves back in the depth of their despair. Unfortunately, this is a normal aspect of the grieving process. This is also where a good support system helps to keep the griever from losing hope and to buoy their spirits and face the fight for another day.

Neither style is right or wrong. Both styles are effective. What style of griever are you? Joanne is a combination of both. For example, she took on the leadership of the Brain Injury Hope Foundation (a 21-year-old non-profit organization) with her business partner in addition to their consulting business while dealing with the acute effects of brain injury due to the loss of her partner. Being actively involved in both businesses enabled Joanne to feel a sense of reward, which was incredibly healing, and her work was of great support during a very trying time. Self-care became even more important throughout this process.

Self-Care Techniques

Self-care is imperative as you deal with the anguish, anger, and loneliness that one experiences during the grieving process. Well intentioned self-care can lead to acceptance and acquaintance with yourself as your own best friend. Self-care looks different to different people and is as unique to the person as a brain injury is unique to the survivor.

It is imperative to choose to take care of yourself at this most vulnerable time. Grieving your brain injury or injuries is like being in a foreign country—take your time. Embrace all aspects you encounter. Don't rush the emotional part. Slow down and take care of yourself like you've never done before as you align your cognitive and emotional beings.

Self-care includes going to the doctor for regular checkups and to properly manage medications (if this pertains to you), as well as for annual wellness exams.

Self-care also includes resting, eating nutritious meals, sticking to a regular sleep routine, drinking plenty of water, and engaging in exercise (swimming, walking, jogging, weight training, yoga, tai chi, etc.). Get a massage, do body work, watch movies that make you happy and laugh, engage in the expressive arts, listen to music that calms you and your brain—or just go outside, put your feet in the grass, look up to the sky, and howl like a wolf at the moon!

Short on time? Here's a list of 10 to 15 minute self-care ideas:

- Hold or play with a pet.

- Take a walk around the block.

- Play a quick game online.

- Eat lunch outside on the grass.

- Write three things daily that you're grateful for—shift to an attitude of gratitude!

- Massage your feet, rolling on a tennis ball or rolling pin.

- Find a reason to laugh.

- Listen to soothing music.

- Help someone in need (this may take more than 15 minutes!).

- Keep a journal.

- Mindfully observe a flower, sunshine, the blue sky, and other beauty around you.

- Do a random act of kindness.

- Inhale calming essential oils.

- Take a nap.

- Exercise or dance like no one is watching.

- Cry, yell, or scream in your car.

- Take a coffee or tea break.

- Take 10 deep breaths.

Slow down. Give yourself a chance to go in and out of grief. Give yourself permission to be where you are. Your body, mind, and soul are in a different position than where they were before. If your body wants to rest, then *rest!*

Honor yourself; give yourself me time making sure to put yourself on your to do list and on your calendar. Make yourself a priority. Take a pajama day—set aside a day to stay in your pajamas, hang out, take a bath, watch positive television shows (or whatever helps you relax), chill out, and go offline.

If you love animals and you are not allergic, a pet is a fabulous support system that helps with self-care. Pets are a comfort and make you feel as though you are not alone. They love unconditionally, are like family, and help bridge the gap between feeling isolated and alone and feeling as though you matter. Pets step in to help you through your many daily challenges. Joanne's cat, Brie, has been an incredible comfort to her and has helped tremendously with her grieving process by offering unconditional love, being a positive energy in her home, and creating much love and joy.

Another aspect of self-care is self-advocacy. As mentioned in Chapter 3, advocate for yourself and/or find someone who will be your advocate. According to George Henry Lewis, "The only cure for grief is action."[8] Your life has changed, and the capacity you had to advocate for yourself may have also changed. Accept and embrace the new you—the transformation that happens through grieving a traumatic experience—with the help and support of others. If you do not have others in your life who can advocate for you, find a support group of like-minded individuals who understand and can be empathetic and compassionate with you.

Select people you can be genuine with. Be yourself—whoever you are in the moment. Grief challenges the world the way you knew and viewed it. You are not in control as much as you might think you are, and therefore might not feel as safe in the world as you did before.

Learn to set boundaries in a way you never had to before because of your vulnerability and raw emotions. Practice saying no to the demands and requests of others. When you do make a plan, give yourself an out in case you do not have the energy or emotional capacity to go through it—or you just do not feel like it when the time comes.

When you're having a good day, it is okay to educate others. When you are having a bad day, it is okay not to care. It is okay not to care about what others feel. It's not your job to make people comfortable or feel good. Give yourself permission to set boundaries, take care of yourself, and do what's best for you in this present moment. When your reserves are depleted and you don't have the energy, it is okay to *not* want to make it okay for others. It's your job to take care of yourself in each and every moment.

Know that any anger that arises from grieving one or more brain injuries is normal. What you do with that anger is imperative to your moving forward. We suggest working with a grief counselor or therapist. Grief counseling helps you walk down the hallway to a new normal. We also suggest reading (or listening to) grief books that support your process and progress.

The good news is that as human beings, we are very good at adapting and adjusting as time moves forward. We are and can be resilient. Be proactive as you manage your self-care. Be kind and gentle with yourself as you go through the grieving process.

How to Help Others Support You with Your Brain Injury: A Baker's Dozen

1. Tell others that silence could be just what you need. Let them know that saying nothing rather than offering clichés can bring comfort, that just their presence is enough at times. Tell them they could squeeze your hand or give you a hug or just *listen*. This could mean more than ill-chosen words that could be discounting.

2. Ask others to call often and check in, especially in the beginning and for many months thereafter. Let them know they shouldn't expect you to call them since your energy level may be low and you may not remember things easily. Ask them to please understand if you need to cut the conversation short.

3. If friends/family ask what they can do for you, ask them to bring food, go for walks with you, and invite you to dinner and other social outings. Let them know that you may or may not accept an

invitation depending upon how you are feeling on that particular day.

4. Offer a specific date and time to engage in an activity when you're usually the least fatigued and have the most energy.

5. Ask others to be patient with you if you decide not to do things with them right away or for many months. Ask them to stay the course with you, if possible.

6. Tell others that it is okay to ask how you are doing and what is going on with your brain injury, if that's the case for you.

7. Ask others to be patient with you as you navigate this new life of yours that you didn't want but have to figure out. Ask them to practice patience if you repeat yourself, forget or lose things, or switch moods.

8. Ask others to avoid pitying you. Ask them to care about you.

9. Ask others to be forgiving if you are insensitive to their problems at this time. Let them know that you're like an empty vessel; you feel drained and depleted with nothing left to give. Again, ask for their patience.

10. Ask others for their understanding if you turn a deaf ear to criticism at this time. If they must offer criticism, ask them to give it lovingly and compassionately.

11. Tell others not to expect you to be the same as you were before. Let them know you are a different person and you have been through a traumatic experience. Ask them to please accept you for who you are today.

12. Tell others to avoid trying to fix you. Tell them that sometimes you just need a shoulder to cry on or to vent.

13. When you are faced with suggestions from others and/or feel discounted, consider responding, *I know you mean well and care about my well-*

being, and at this time in my life I do not need any suggestions. Please don't be offended, as I'm speaking my truth with compassion.

A Final Note

Learn to integrate the loss into your life. You are never done, and you never stop grieving. You're never done, because you're never the same. Traumatic experiences change you forever. You have a choice to stay in the negativity of it or move forward in a more positive way.

You transform yourself by taking your traumatic experience and turning it into a purpose—helping others through their own lemons in life. Helping others *is* helping you.

When you are grieving, time doesn't necessarily heal your pain; it's what you do with your time while grieving that makes a difference. Brain injury also isn't about time; it's what you do with it. Joanne's heart cracked wide open, opening up for her the possibility for love, growth, and compassion for herself and for others. The expectation of grieving the loss of her loved one and working through her brain injuries helped her transform the expectation of herself and others.

As mentioned, grief isn't an event, it's a process. Going through the grieving process affects everything and screams vulnerability. This process is important so address your grief. Don't expect grief to disappear just because you're not thinking about it. If you try to ignore it, it'll come out in a different way and could lead to unwanted emotional and health issues.

Release your grief with love and gratitude. Some days, you may feel as though you're on top of the world; other days you may feel as though you're in the eye of the storm. You may also feel everything in between.

As you go through the grief process, you'll learn to create a different relationship with yourself in a different way. "Grief can be the garden of compassion. If you keep your heart open through everything your pain can become your greatest ally in your life's search for love and wisdom."
Rumi

My mission in life is not merely to survive, but to thrive; and to do so with some passion, some compassion, some humor, and some style.

Maya Angelou

Chapter 8 Epilogue: Where I Am Today

In the Addendum you will be able to read letters about an extremely vulnerable time in my life after three rear-end accidents that occurred within a four-month time period and the ramifications of those accidents on my behavior, moods, collegial relationships, personal relationships, business partners, and friends. That was then and this is now.

You also read about the lessons I learned along the way as I moved beyond the physical and emotional trauma of getting hit and dealing with litigation and grief. I looked back through my rearview mirror to reflect and assess those years and share lessons learned. Hopefully, what you have read will resonate and you will find it helpful.

Today, I am happy to report that I am, once again, thriving. It has taken patience, perseverance, incredible support teams, an intention to get better and have a life worth living, and time to get here. Gratitude has been a big part of why I am thriving. I am grateful to be able to participate in my life work with CTAT, LLC, Brain Injury Hope Foundation, and the brain injury Survivor Series. I am grateful for my family and friends who have stuck by me, no matter what. I am grateful to have wonderful bodyworkers who help me manage chronic pain. I am grateful for spiritual teachings. I am grateful for the recreation center where I swim frequently for the good of my body, mind, and spirit. I am grateful to have my cat, Brie, who loves me and is good company.

Life happens. Sometimes it is a series of curveballs or setbacks that cause us to barely survive. Then we learn to not only survive but to thrive! In this time of thriving, I still experience exhaustion, cognitive fatigue (I am highly functioning until I am not), and chronic body pain. I have learned ways to compensate, using self-care techniques, going to health practitioners, and swimming to keep my body moving and my spirit soaring.

I have learned to make adjustments, to adapt from who I was to who I have become. I have learned to live with a new reality, accepting what is and what isn't, and it has truly been profound. I know, *really* know, how precious life is and how important it is to do things on the bucket list while I am able to do so.

We are a work in progress. I believe, no matter what anyone tells us, that we can improve, and there is no time stamp on that improvement. Today's evolving avenues of support include new technologies, breakthrough brain research, and innovative treatments.

In closing, I encourage you to listen to one of my favorite songs. It is a vision for what I wish for all of us. The song is called "Bring It On" by Jana Stanfield and it moved me. I thought of the brain injury community and anyone who grieves the loss of a loved one. What is meaningful about this song is that it depicts the yearning to move forward while accepting where you are now. It helps you embrace the fact that your life as it was is never going to be the same. So, embrace your new life as it is now and celebrate it.

Getting Hit, Getting Up, Moving Beyond…

Here's to surviving…

Here's to **thriving**…

Here's to YOU!

Addendum

Sometimes, people look at me and think I'm doing great. There are several letters in the Addendum that show what a difficult journey this has been. Rebecca, my attorney, asked people to write these letters to show the changes that occurred after the three accidents in 2014. My friends and colleagues were asked to write honest letters. When they gave me the letters to read, they said they were afraid of what I might think when I read them. I said, "Please give the letters to me, because it shows me where I was and the progress I've made. I am not there now."

Joanne McLain Statement

Changes I have noticed about Joanne Cohen since May 2014. I have worked as a colleague with Joanne Cohen on a variety of projects for the past several years. I was aware that she was a long-term survivor of a traumatic brain injury and recognized occasional symptoms like difficulty remembering tasks when she was tired, but those symptoms appeared to be mild and she managed them well through behavioral strategies and reminders she had learned to utilize. Generally, it seemed that those strategies functioned more as insurance that she wouldn't forget important details and, most of the time, she did not need to rely on them much.

I am a Licensed Professional Counselor and have some experience in evaluating and counseling survivors of traumatic brain injuries, so I can recognize when Joanne Cohen is displaying symptoms consistent with such injuries. Before her first accident in 2014, her symptoms were present but minor and she had excellent adaptive skills. She was also clearly an intelligent, outgoing, energetic, positive person who was usually focused on achieving results while consistently sensitive to other people's feelings and needs. I would describe her energy level and ability to focus on projects as above average. Her ability to problem solve and consider the relative importance of details was similarly high. She was able to avoid distractions and sustain her focus on a project for multiple hours. Her vocabulary was appropriately complex and precise for a professional position and her verbal fluency was generally impressive, although she would show some moderate signs of delay in word retrieval from fatigue by the end of a long day. She generally preferred to maintain routines that facilitated her memory but was able to operate well when circumstances deviated from that routine and she functioned very well as a professional in a complex, demanding position.

After her first accident in 2014, she initially showed significant effects of pain and muscle stiffness, especially in her neck and jaw. She had difficulty holding her neck in a straight position and would frequently ask me to sit directly across the table from her rather than at an angle, which would exacerbate her neck pain. She fatigued easily and had difficulty staying focused on a project. She reported feeling tired and dispirited frequently, which was a significant departure from her previous behavior. She would forget appointments (which she never did prior to the accidents) and was particularly upset when she forgot a phone meeting with an important client, a lapse I had never seen in her prior to May 2014. Joanne has a significant talent for nurturing relationships and places a high value on customer service, so she would normally prioritize a scheduled meeting with a client.

More than once I saw her look at notes in her own handwriting that she said were not familiar to her, which I had never observed before May 2014. She began to forget tasks that she had agreed to do, sometimes not even remembering that she had said she would do that task. She had significant difficulty in reading for comprehension, sometimes needing to ask others about the point of a written statement and she sometimes avoided reading longer passages. She would repeat statements and questions she had already asked and gotten answered. She would sometimes perseverate on particular details of a project beyond the point were other people had moved on to other details. Prior to her accidents, she would have been sensitive to the social situation and close off the prior subject in order to move on.

One of the most concerning changes I witnessed in her was her difficulty in maintaining a positive attitude, which had been one of her shining strengths. She became more irritable and made frequent nervous movements such as shifting her sitting position, touching her neck and hair, and rearranging papers. Prior to her accidents she displayed a high energy level but moved her body in a more relaxed fashion. She worried almost to the point of obsession about any lapse in her thinking processes or memory, asking repeatedly what I noticed about the lapses. Instead of the bright, charming and outgoing woman that she had been before the accidents, Joanne became more reclusive, felt uncomfortable in group situations and withdrew more from the team she had enjoyed working with before. It was clear that she was managing to maintain an adequate performance of her work duties because of her intelligence, prior training for coping with traumatic brain injury and sheer force of will, but that maintenance was taking a hard toll on her. She was told by professionals that she should take time off to rest and recover but she found that difficult due to the demands of her professional position and her own work ethic so she continued to maintain a nearly full-time work schedule despite multiple appointments for assessment and treatment of her symptoms.

As of March 2015, Joanne seems to have gradually recovered much of her prior abilities, due in large part to her drive to improve herself and what appears to be excellent care she is receiving, but she still has more difficulties than before the accidents. She still tires easily and has more difficulty with short-term memory and word retrieval than she had prior to May 2014. It is clear that she still suffers from headaches and pain in her neck, and her movements are still somewhat stiff. She is able to focus more consistently and for longer periods of time but still shows difficulties when she is stressed or tired.

She holds herself to a high standard and has been putting a tremendous amount of effort into her recovery, so I am certain that she will continue to improve, but it has been at a high emotional and mental cost for her (not to mention the monetary cost and loss of time to appointments, driving and skills practice).

If there are other observations or insights I can provide, please feel free to ask.

Gayann Brandenburg Statement

I have been Joanne Cohen's supervisor for almost five years. This letter is to describe the changes I have seen in Joanne's work performance since three car accidents she has recently experienced.

Joanne has very high expectations of herself and is a very motivated person in general. She definitely is frustrated with her current situation and its impact on her work performance.

Joanne's stamina has decreased. She fatigues after more complex tasks and it can take her several days to feel re-energized. This results in her having reduced productivity during those days.

Her fatigue is also related to her chronic pain. She is often in pain, especially her neck and back, and has needed accommodations to adjust her work station. Chronic pain equals exhaustion.

Joanne's ability to work on complex tasks (executive functioning such as strategizing, making decisions, planning and organizing) has diminished and is even worse when she is fatigued. She is not able to easily divide her attention. These tasks will now take her longer, she is more likely to make mistakes and need assistance in double checking her work, and these tasks drain Joanne's energy, as mentioned above.

Joanne also has experienced more issues with memory, especially short-term retrieval. She has forgotten meetings, conversations, where she has placed documents, and simple routine things like completing her time card. She needs additional support to stay organized and remember things.

Joanne's emotions have been impacted by these recent events also. Because she is not operating at what she considers peak performance, she can lack self-confidence, be very hard on herself, and need re-assurance that she is a valued employee. She also has lower frustration tolerance, and can easily be frustrated with co-worker interactions, or even noise and over-stimulation. For example, Joanne came to the company holiday party and the crowd, the crowd noise and all the activity overwhelmed her to the point she could not stay at the party. Normally

Joanne is a very social person and would have totally participated and enjoyed the party. Another example is a department retreat that was held this summer. Joanne became very sensitive after receiving feedback from a colleague and shut down. She was emotional, had trouble participating in the rest of the retreat, became sensitive about a cooking competition, and overall had a very difficult time in what would have typically been a very enjoyable day for her.

Joanne has done everything she can to improve her functioning – testing, cognitive therapy, PT, vision testing and new glasses for computer work, etc. She is usually able to flex her schedule to make these appointments, but they are also exhausting. She is a very valued employee and I hope she can continue to get the support she needs.

Linda Fankboner Statement

I have been close friends with Joanne Cohen for 24 years, and have always known her to be a high-energy, driven, enthusiastic, persevering person who was very organized, and with her energetic nature, always completed tasks and obligations on time. She was critically injured in a head-on traffic accident while vacationing in the Bahamas in 1992. In addition to a broken hip and multiple broken bones, she also suffered a Traumatic Brain Injury (TBI). She went through years of physical therapy, occupational therapy, and intensive cognitive brain therapies. She worked diligently to heal herself from this terrible tragedy.

And then May, June and August of 2014 happened, where she was rear-ended in three different months, in three separate accidents, by three different drivers. Much of the healing that Joanne had worked so hard to achieve was sent into a tailspin and she suffered a severe setback. The whiplash she experienced in each of these rear-ends greatly exacerbated the neck injury and TBI she sustained in 1992. She experiences headaches and constant pain on a daily basis.

Before these three accidents, Joanne was independent, free-wheeling, socially active, highly energetic and on top of her game. We have shared many experiences of friendship over the past 24 years—sharing dinners and gifts at our annual birthdays and at holiday time; she was always ebullient, energetic, jovial, and enthusiastic. She has many friends and regularly would socialize with them at dinners, concerts, parties and many social events. She entertained almost weekly with dinner parties in her home. She loved to travel, and also loved to swim at her local gym. In other words, she lived a robust, full, happy and engaging life with her partner and many friends.

But since these accidents last summer, she has retreated from a lot of social activities and isolates herself more than she used to. I have noticed definite changes in Joanne's behavior, especially in two areas—lack of energy and forgetfulness. There have been several instances where I have called her on the telephone, and she has answered with a lethargic, low level of energy; when I commented that she seemed "not her usual self," she answered that she "was just exhausted, and was not sleeping well at all." She and I had made plans to go to two different movies in the last month, and said we'd go out for a bite to eat after the movie. When the movies ended (both times), Joanne said to me, "I'm sorry but I just don't feel like going out to eat…I'm too tired and just need to go home." Heretofore, she always was game to go out to dinner after a movie. This was a definite departure from her old self. She has said several times in our phone conversations that she doesn't entertain at home near as much as she used to, nor accepts as many dinner invitations with friends, because she's "just too tired and feels chronically fatigued."

As to forgetfulness and short-term memory loss, I have noticed several instances where she just forgot or didn't remember. For example, we went to a movie last September at a huge AMC 24-movie theatre near her neighborhood. Just recently, we talked about seeing one of the Oscar-nominated movies together, and she said, "You should come out and see the beautiful AMC theatre with the most incredibly comfortable seats." And I said, "Yes, I know, we went to a movie their last fall." And she said, "Oh, I didn't remember. I forgot that we went there." This has happened on several occasions. She lives by post-a-notes that she sticks everywhere to help her remember things we've discussed, or things we've made plans for.

There is no judgment here, only compassion and complete understanding, for what Joanne is going through. As a close friend, I know the real Joanne—fun loving, intelligent, hardworking, effervescent, energetic, and she had a keen memory prior to last summer's accidents. She is a genuine optimist, and in spite of these cognitive deficits, she still remains optimistic and hardworking, but nothing flows as easily as it used to.... these accidents have definitely set her back, cognitively, physically and mentally.

Life is not always fair, but I believe it is just, and I hope justice will be given to Joanne Cohen. As her life-long friend, I support her unconditionally.

If you have any questions, please don't hesitate to call me at the number above.

James Dunn Statement

I've written this letter to describe the personal and professional changes I observed in Joanne Cohen following three car accidents in which she was rear-ended during the summer of 2014. I've known

Joanne since 2007 and have worked with her on and off over that time; therefore, I have an informed baseline for describing the impacts I've perceived since the accidents.

Joanne was hired by Policy Studies Inc. (PSI) in 2007 as an executive coach to design and implement a leadership development program for the company, which anticipated rapid growth. As part of the Leadership Pipeline Program, Joanne worked with PSI's executives to identify those competencies (e.g., driving for results, coaching, decision making, and emotional intelligence, among others) they believed would be most essential in the leaders they would require to grow. The program was designed to identify and strengthen those abilities in high-potential employees identified by executive management. As the head of marketing, my team worked closely with Joanne to develop communications materials for the program; consequently, I gained great insight and appreciation at the deliberation and expertise that Joanne put into the design for the program.

I was privileged to be among the first round of employees selected to participate in the program. I was thoroughly impressed by the sophistication and thoroughness of the program as well as how specific and insightful the coaching was for me. I definitely credit much of my career success since then to the skills and self-awareness that I learned from Joanne. More importantly, her work among my peers in the program created a strong, cohesive and effective senior leadership team for the Company. Looking back, I know that Joanne worked quietly behind the scenes — taking people aside to privately discuss her observations and concerns about interactions that weren't going as well as they should.

When she left the PSI to pursue another opportunity in 2009, many remained in touch with Joanne and sought out her thoughts and insights as we moved forward in our careers. She also sought out my advice when she was at Rocky Mountain Human Services regarding branding and messaging for one of that company's service offerings. Joanne is generous with her time and an awesome collaborator.

In my role as Director of Marketing for MAXIMUS, I was asked to identify options for training high-level leaders in the Human Services North America division of our Company. The President of the division was concerned that her team wasn't effective when presenting opportunities to the Company's Business Review Committee (BRC), comprising the CEO, CFO, and President among others. Specifically, they became rattled by the format of the meeting, which most resembles an episode of Shark Tank in which budding entrepreneurs present their ideas to five titans of industry and attempt to convince one of them to invest in their idea. I turned to Joanne who was Senior Consultant at CTAT / Rocky Mountain Human Services. She developed an Articulate Leader program that comprised one day of classroom time, one- day of taped presentations and group feedback sessions, and one month later we held a Mock BRC with each of the President's direct reports taking the role of a BRC member. We saw a significant improvement in the participant's confidence levels and ability to respond to questions while maintaining the story line of their presentation. The participants told us this had been the best and most valuable training they'd experienced, and many have continued to contact Joanne for individual coaching sessions. The President also noted a significant improvement in how BRC presentations were received by the Company's executives.

We've since amended Joanne's original contract 15 times to add additional training and executive coaching services. These have included Raising the Bar workshops at three program sites to help the site's management team overcome dysfunctions among the team's members and improve performance.

During the summer of 2014, Joanne was rear-ended in three separate accidents. Since then, my colleagues and I have noted the following changes, which we've had to accommodate:

She's physically weaker and requires far more assistance when traveling or setting up training rooms, which is why she generally asks to fly on the same flights that I do when we're going to a different Company location.

She tires far more quickly and has difficulty maintaining her usual high-energy classroom style for full-day sessions. Fatigue was also a factor during a 1.5-day workshop we asked her to facilitate for the President's leadership team in Miami. The first exercise focused on Strengths Finder 2.0, which was effective and intensive for the group. She then began working on Emotional Intelligence, which bombed. She didn't have a process for facilitating it, which is very unlike her, and then it's as if she shut down and couldn't think. We called for a break so that Joanne could regroup and finish out the session.

She's not as detailed as she had been. For this reason, I've had my team assist her in reworking charts and course materials—particularly charts reporting out the results of testing she's asked participants to take—to ensure they're accurate and presented clearly.

Her short-term memory seems to have been impacted. Consequently, she's adjusted by writing frequent emails and making frequent calls to me and others at MAXIMUS as various ideas or concerns come to her. Prior to the accident, she did a much better job setting touch base appointments to run through a punch list of issues she'd identified since the prior meeting. As the project manager responsible for her contract, I am having to make an extra effort to keep our contract amendments and billing straight.

We greatly value our working relationship with Joanne and continue to turn to her for her exceptional insights, training and coaching services. That's why we are accommodating some of her current weaknesses as we see her working hard to recover from her injuries. I do know she's really pushing herself very hard to keep up with our service needs at the level we need, which I respect and admire.

Roni Baker Statement

To introduce myself, my name is Roni Baker and I am the partner to Joanne Cohen. Joanne and I met in 1995 and have been together for almost 20 years.

Joanne has always been a go getter. Joanne is very active in not only in the business environment but the social arena as well. Our calendar is always busy for dinners, business functions, weekend trips, movies, and dinner parties. Weekends are always full of new adventures.

Joanne is an English Major and we do have fun in Joanne correcting my verbiage and pronunciation on words.

Joanne's health has always been good, and I always felt fortunate that, unlike my associates who are either sick most of the time or complained about their health.

Joanne is admired throughout Colorado on her speaking engagements. She is always invited to be on a panel, speak on a specific topic, introductions, and her company is complimented throughout their network on her speaking appointments.

Joanne's demeanor with me is always with a ring in her voice.

Joanne has a lot of respect for time. She is always either a little early or right on time. Yes, this *was* Joanne.

Since these three accidents there has been a great change.

After the first accident her body started having body and face pains.

After the second accident her body was really having pains, again both body and face. After the third accident, Joanne lost the sparkle in her eyes.

Situation changes that I have found:

Our calendar is sparse. She is very tired now and does not participate in loud active engagements.

Dinners out are almost nil.

Weekends are for body therapy.

Joanne finds it difficult at times to find the words she wants to express.

Joanne speaks in left field sometime, i.e., instead of saying 45 miles per hour, 45 % per hour.

Joanne continually has headaches, her teeth hurt, her jaw hurts, her neck hurts, and her shoulders hurt.

Joanne limits any speaking engagements. Those projects with work, it takes longer for her to put together the materials.

Joanne has started to be late to functions, not realizing that it's time to leave.

Joanne is leaving her credit cards (3 times) at stores.

Joanne is leaving her coat at restaurants.

Joanne is forgetting that she put her glasses in her purse.

Joanne has flooded the basement because she forgot that the water was running in the laundry room.

Closeness is not inviting anymore.

A lot of snappiness in her voice.

Effort is taken for whatever we decide to do.

The sparkle is gone from her eyes.

I appreciate the opportunity to express my feelings on how Joanne and I interact. Please do not hesitate to call me for any further questions or inquiries. Sincerely,
Roni Baker

On a more positive note, this is an article written by a colleague and friend of Joanne's in 2010:

Extra Ordinary People[9]

By Melanie Mulhall

Later she would say that the evening she wrote all of those checks, amounting to tens of thousands of dollars, was one of the most joyful and fulfilling evenings of her life. She smiled a Madonna-like smile of remembrance as she told me about it, more than a decade later.

Joanne had suffered life-changing injuries, while on vacation in the Bahamas. She had planned the vacation because she was burned out. She felt that her life was not working and that she was not walking her talk. She needed a break.

She got it. Actually, she suffered several breaks: a massive hip injury, fractured pelvis, and closed-head injury. Sitting in a vehicle, stopped next to a curb, she was hit head on by a truck going 65 miles an hour. During the 24-hour ordeal of being air ambulanced back to the United States, the 3 ½ weeks in the hospital (two of which were spent in traction), and a year of physical therapy, Joanne had to remind herself frequently that she was lucky to be alive.

Joanne's auto insurance did not cover her outside of the United States and the complexities involved with the resolution of her insurance claim were compounded by the necessity of navigating Bahamian bureaucracy. Two and a half years after the accident, she finally had a settlement check.

Her expenses during the 2 ½ year period of the time might have discouraged another person to the point of bankruptcy. Not Joanne. Doctors, physical therapists, friends, family, and other kind souls had all deferred payment services rendered and money loaned.

Joanne had an admirable support system. She also had an admirable mindset. I doubt that it ever occurred to Joanne to default on her outstanding debts, because a person who defaults on her debts is not how Joanne sees herself. In fact, I know exactly what Joanne said: "This is not the truth about me."

This mindset of holding firm to the vision of the version of herself she chose to live out also resulted in her doctors telling her that she had a normal hip, four years after proclaiming that her hip would never be the same – despite surgery and physical therapy. Joanne's ability to hold a vision of herself as healed and whole had as much to do with her healing as the medical treatment.

The same mindset led Joanne to the night she wrote checks, smiling and blessing each one as she signed it. In my mind, Joanne's life is one of heroic proportions and Joanne, herself, is a heroine. She is not a mythological heroine; she is a flesh and blood, everyday heroine.

Joanne is not alone. Everyday heroes and heroines abound. They live next door to us…or with us. They come from every walk of life and practice every profession.

Endnotes

[1] https://dojos.info/WayOfTheCrane

[2] Acimovic, Mary Lou. Mild Traumatic Brain Injury: The Guidebook (2010).

[3] Therrien, Jeffrey, (2013). "The Other Side of the Fence" letter written on September 13, 2013.

[4] Carl Sandburg Quotes. BrainyQuote.com. Brainy Media Inc, 2019. 23 March 2019. https://www.brainyquote.com/quotes/carl_sandburg_345254

[5] Nouwen, Henri (1988) "Road to Daybreak"

[6] Worden, William J. "Four Tasks of Mourning." See https://whatsyourgrief.com/wordens-four-tasks-of-mourning

[7] See https://whatsyourgrief.com/grief-and-gender-a-preamble

[8] Lewis, George Henry. See https://www.dictionary-quotes.com/the-only-cure-for-grief-is-action-george-henry-lewis

[9] Mulhall, M. (May - June 2005). "Extraordinary Ordinary People" Published in Enlightened Woman Magazine, p. 20.

About the Author

Joanne E. Cohen has over 37 years combined experience in coaching, consulting, organization development, facilitation, and training. She has consulted, trained and coached executives and their

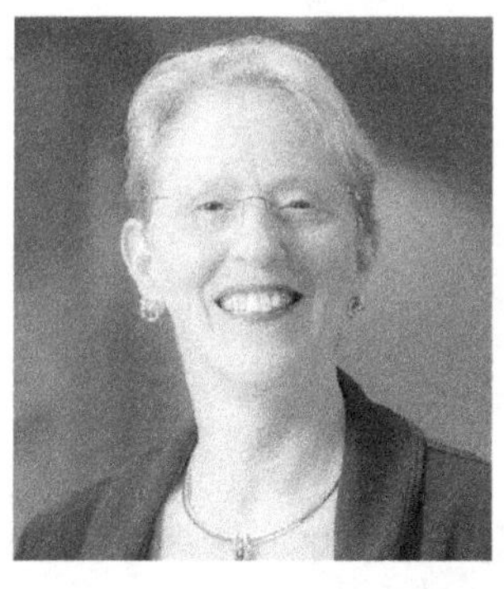

teams in the planning and implementation of new strategic directions that are in alignment with the business goals and objectives of their companies. In addition, Joanne designed and implemented a highly successful corporate Leadership Pipeline Program with limited funding. She currently consults, coaches and facilitates sessions with leadership and front-line teams for a major $2.4 billion company's Human Services, Corporate Training, and Health Divisions, in addition to many other clients. Joanne has demonstrated exemplary professional presentation skills. She has kept pace with the current business needs and provides clients with excellent resources for understanding leadership, and managing change and stress. Her expertise domestically and globally spans the health and human services, telecommunications, hi-tech, manufacturing, mining, biomedical, oil and gas, and aerospace industries in addition to teaching Higher Education classes.

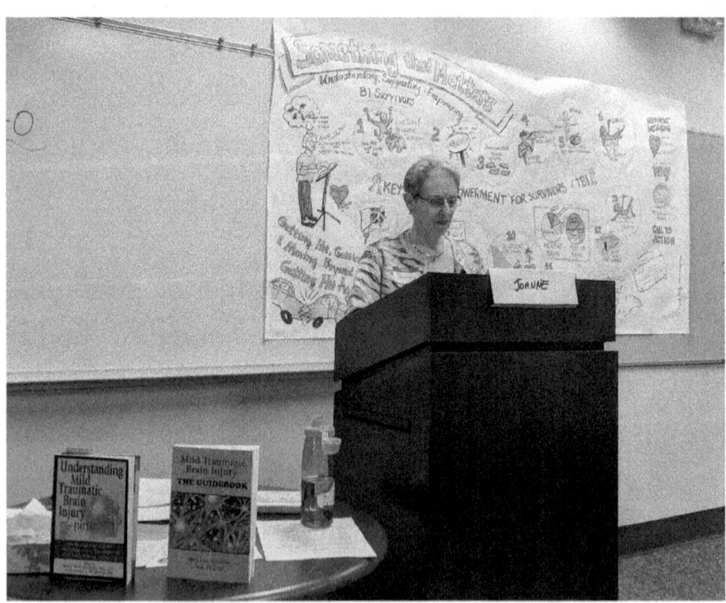

Joanne presenting at a Brain Injury Survivor Series. She announced her intention to write this book during this program.

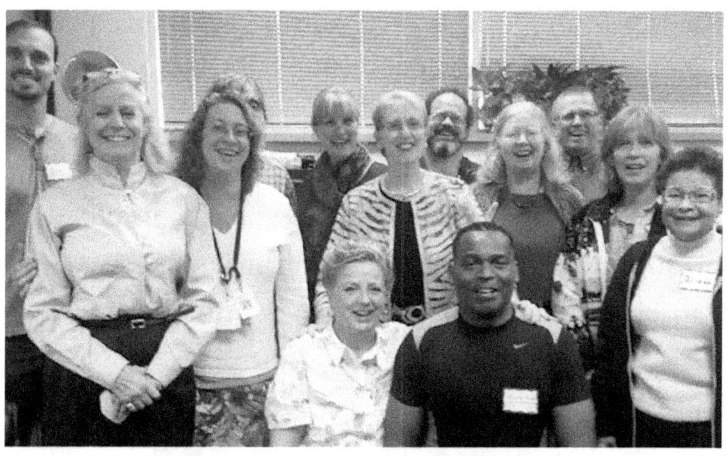

A group of brain injury survivors and
professionals celebrating thriving.

Joanne is a Traumatic Brain Injury survivor after having
one major automobile accident and three subsequent
accidents. She has learned many coping skills over the
years. She joined CTAT at Rocky Mountain Human
Services in 2010 and is currently a Managing Partner for
CTAT, LLC (Coaching, Training, and Transformation)
as well as Vice-President of the Brain Injury Hope
Foundation (BIHF), a non-profit organization that
serves people with Traumatic Brain Injuries (TBI)
by providing emergency funds and training. She
designs and facilitates the BIHF Survivor Series for
TBI survivors, family members, friends, caregivers,
and professionals who serve this community and is

passionate about these grant-funded programs. Joanne was the liaison for the National Engaging Veterans with Disabilities in National and Community Service projects. She speaks at conferences as a Keynote Speaker as well as for breakout sessions, consults with organizations to support critical business issues, and participates in various other grants/initiatives.

On a more personal note, Joanne meets with various groups of friends monthly, loves to swim laps, enjoys movies, music, plays, spirituality, dining out, and entertaining; is a self-proclaimed foodie who likes to have dinner parties at home for friends and she loves pizza, wine and dark chocolate.

Joanne lives in Colorado with her cat Brie.

Speaking, Coaching, and Training Engagements

If you would like to engage Joanne as a Keynote Speaker, Panelist, or for a workshop; for Trial Coaching and Consulting for expert witnesses and/or clients; for consulting regarding how to set up a Brain Injury Survivor Series in your location; or for Leadership Development Workshops, Team Building Webinars, and/or Coaching; please visit braininjuryhopefoundation.org or ctatllc.com for more information and/or call 844-444-4522.

Rave Reviews for Survivor Series

"The panel was awesome and had great personal stories to share and connect with…so much wisdom and compassion—thank you so much!"

"Everyone in this room had their hearts connected several times and this leads to acceptance!"

"I liked being with my tribe!...I liked survivors sharing with each other...This is the first time I have felt that the people have walked in my shoes...I don't feel alone for the first time since my injury 3.5 years ago."

"Thanks for paying attention and sharing what people need."

"Joanne's questions and monitoring the panels and moving the conversations forward were excellent."

Rave Reviews for
The Articulate Leader Program

"We've used The Articulate Leader Program to prepare our up-and-coming leaders to have greater visibility and credibility with clients and executive management. I've been truly impressed with the advances I've seen in their performance as they present with greater clarity and confidence."

Division President, US Human Services, MAXIMUS

"The Articulate Leader class was a highly valuable program that added to my skills and confidence in presenting. Joanne and the supporting executive team provided thorough content that covered every aspect of presenting and provided me with tools to make my presentations more engaging, more informative, and to help manage the nerves that I inevitably experience before major presentations. This class really pushed me out of my comfort zone, forcing me to look at a comprehensive view of my project and learning to prepare for and answer tough questions. It was clear that Joanne was fully prepared, anticipating the needs of each participant. The class was deeply engaged in listening to every presentation because the tools allowed each of us to prepare interesting and valuable content and present it effectively. I understand much more about executive expectations and myself that I did when I began. Thanks to Joanne and the team for an excellent and valuable course."

Participant, January- February 2019 Class

Rave Reviews for Raising the Bar Workshops

"It is incredibly apparent that leadership and the topics surrounding Joanne's lifework and it is a pleasure seeing the joy it brings her."

"The tools, resources, book references, etc. are invaluable in moving forward to create a team that walks and talks in synch. This class designed and facilitated by Joanne is a great compilation of leadership skills, tools, and techniques. I loved everything!"

"The training was very relevant to my day-to-day job and provided many tools for me to grow as a Leader and personally. I truly appreciate Joanne's time and her dedication to the training! Thank you."

"I enjoyed the program and feel that the takeaways from this training can be applied to so many aspects of my life."

"This is one of the most powerful trainings I have experienced. We focused on the positives and easily tackled our to do list. I appreciate Joanne's feedback and really look forward to implementing her tips and tools."

"The tools gained from the program will assist in work and home. I look forward to watching them work their magic."

"The energy I brought home after the first day of the workshop allowed me a better understanding about my personal relationships."

"This class helped me gain a new perspective and strengthened the positive relationships with my co-workers."

"Raising the Bar helped me understand my leadership team and what problems/struggles they face. This will not only help me communicate with them, but to help meet their needs."

"I have been implementing the problem-solving model tool. I used the super hero pose today while preparing, and overall, loved the program! Can't wait to follow up in 6 months."

"This class was a great experience, not just applicable to work, but to my personal life. This was a much-needed training to assist our leadership team with refining our vision and assisting us to develop a positive game plan to raise the bar."

"Great, a once in a lifetime opportunity!"

Rave Reviews for Coaching

"I worked with Joanne for over 6 months. Her coaching was the reason that I am now a Vice President. Joanne showed me and helped me overcome the multitude of issues I had as a Director in dealing with people. Her coaching showed me that the issues were with me and opened my eyes to different ways to deal with people of all levels in our division and company. Without Joanne's guidance and coaching I would not have succeeded in my career without her."

P. Baylinson
Vice President, US Health & Human Services, MAXIMUS

"In an organization geared toward helping government serve the people, our teams spend an extraordinary amount of time working with individuals who face significant challenges in their lives. As a result, our clients require us to be agile, well informed and articulate. Joanne has been a tremendous asset in helping us to raise the bar with our leadership team, our managers and our projects. From individual coaching sessions to customized team workshops, her fun, yet focused sessions yield results."

Senior Vice President, US Health & Human Services, MAXIMUS

"I have worked with Joanne both personally and professionally for several years. Through Joanne's coaching and mentoring, I have developed into a more confident and capable leader. I have also referred many of my staff to Joanne for coaching and leadership training. Joanne has a keen understanding of human behavior and teaches practical tools to assist with handling the everyday mundane situations to the most challenging personal and professional ones. While maintaining professional boundaries, I have experienced Joanne taking a personal interest in me as her client and appreciate the understanding and compassionate approach she takes to her work. Joanne embodies the sentiment of practice what you preach and her work is truly her life's work."

T. Hinds
Statewide Education and Training Program Director

"Working with Joanne was a catalyst for change in both my personal and professional life. Joanne has a wealth of knowledge and tools available that help to identify and overcome barriers. Her empathy and passion for her work and for each individual she coaches are evident, making it easy to share your challenges and experiences and receive valid, constructive input. Coaching and seminars with Joanne significantly improved my work-life balance and advanced my professional skills. If you bring an open mind and a desire to be the best version of yourself, working with Joanne will absolutely bring about positive change."

M. Royal
Project Manager

Contact Joanne E. Cohen

For more information,

VISIT
braininjuryhopefoundation.org or
ctatllc.com

EMAIL
ctat@ctatllc.com or
jcohen@braininjuryhopefoundation.org

CALL
844-444-4522

9 781733 839709